Temporomandibular Joint - Surgical Reconstruction and Managements

Edited by Raja Kummoona

Published in London, United Kingdom

Temporomandibular Joint - Surgical Reconstruction and Managements
http://dx.doi.org/10.5772/intechopen.98032
Edited by Raja Kummoona

Contributors
Pablo Andrés Crespo Reinoso, Emilio Ruiz Delgado, James Jerez Robalino, Oleg Valentinovich Slesarev, Vladimír Machoň, Michal Beňo, Siddharth Mehta, Kadarkarai Kirupa, R. Rajashri, Kamali Raman, Aishwarya Balaji, Pavithra Elango, Swetha Karupaiah, Leelavathy Gopalakrishnan, Sundaram Ravanasamudram Rajaram, Gauthami Sundar, Rajaram Ravanasamudram Sundaram, Jolanta E. E. Loster, Justyna Grochala, Raja Kummoona

First published in London, United Kingdom, 2023 by IntechOpen
IntechOpen is the global imprint of INTECHOPEN LIMITED, registered in England and Wales, registration number: 11086078, 5 Princes Gate Court, London, SW7 2QJ, United Kingdom

British Library Cataloguing-in-Publication Data
A catalogue record for this book is available from the British Library

Additional hard and PDF copies can be obtained from orders@intechopen.com

Temporomandibular Joint - Surgical Reconstruction and Managements
Edited by Raja Kummoona
p. cm.
Print ISBN 978-1-80355-963-6
Online ISBN 978-1-80355-964-3
eBook (PDF) ISBN 978-1-80355-965-0

Meet the editor

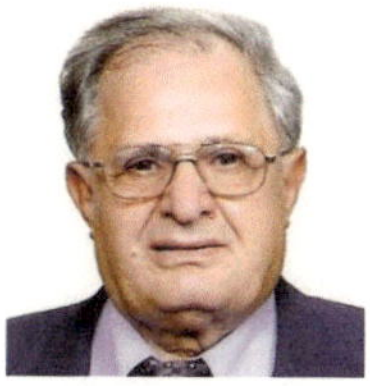

Prof. Raja Kummoona, Emeritus Professor of Maxillofacial Surgery at the Iraqi Board for Medical Specializations, is also a Fellow of the Royal Society of Medicine (FRS), and Fellow of the Royal College of Surgeons (FDSRCS) in the UK. He was a Research Fellow of the Royal College of Surgeons (1975-1977), President of the Iraqi Dental Society (1977-1985), and Registrar of Primary FDSRCS in Iraq (1985-1990). He was awarded the title of most distinguished professor of the University of Baghdad (1991-1992), and was one of the 40 top scientists in Iraq to be awarded a gold medal by the president for 3 years (2000-2002). He has pioneered many TMJ surgical procedures and treatments for maxillofacial injuries, orbit tumors and facial war injuries worldwide. He contributed to research in cancer and developed post-graduate studies in maxillofacial surgery in Iraq. He is the editor of eight books on maxillofacial surgery, he has published 136 original papers in distinguished national and international journals and is a member of the editorial board of 29 international distinguished journals. He is the President of the Iraqi Society of Maxillofacial Surgery, a founder member of the International Society of Head and Neck Trauma, and Founder and former Chairman of the Council of Maxillofacial Surgery, Iraqi Board for Medical Specializations (1993-2010).

Contents

Preface

Temporomandibular Joint - Surgical Reconstruction and Managements brings together the knowledge, skill and experience of a range of experts in the surgical and therapeutic management of the temporomandibular joint (TMJ). Cranio-maxillofacial surgeons have contributed a new understanding of diseases of this unique joint, and researchers are continually working on new techniques for their management.

In this book, we describe the embryology, development and growth of TMJ, together with its anatomy, physiology and growth theories. As well as surgical reconstruction of the TMJ, the book covers recent advances in the management of the most difficult cases of TMJ disease including ankylosis of the TMJ in both adults and children. Other diseases described include first arch syndrome, in which deficient growth and malformation of the face require a series of operations, and condylar hypoplasia, in which an iliac crest graft is used for the restoration of growth, repair and remodeling of the TMJ in children (Kummoona Chondro-Osseous Graft). Subluxation and dislocation, internal derangements of the disc, and recent advances in acute and chronic management of the osteoarthritic disease are also described. Pain in the TMJ and methods of differentiating it from other chronic facial pain are discussed. Diagnostic tools such as an electronic stethoscope for the detection of disc movements, biomechanics of the joint and orthodontic treatments for the correction of the TMJ are also covered.

This book will be useful for neurosurgeons, oral, maxillofacial, craniofacial, and ENT surgeons, and for postgraduate students.

I would like to extend my thanks to Mirena Calmic, Commissioning Editor at IntechOpen, for her kind invitation to edit this volume, to Blanka Gugic, Author Service Manager, for all her efforts, and to everyone who has made this book possible by working on its preparation, printing and publication.

Raja Kummoona
Emeritus Professor of Maxillofacial Surgery,
Iraqi Board for Medical Specializations,
Medical City, Baghdad, Iraq

Section 1

Introduction

Chapter 1

Introductory Chapter: Evolution of the Temporomandibular Joint Surgery

Raja Kummoona

1. Introduction

1.1 History of temporomandibular joint (TMJ) disease and surgery

The temporomandibular joint (TMJ) disease and surgery was known since ancient years. The temporomandibular joint is unique in its development, anatomy, and function and the disease that affect the TMJ rather different from other joints. It consists of two joint cavities one superior and the other inferior in between the articular disc and is covered by synovial fluid that comes from synovial pharynges inside the capsule for lubrication of the TMJ and protein nourishment of the cartilaginous parts of the joint [1, 2].

During the second world war, two great people, Sir Harold Gillies and Sir Kelsy Fry, put the foundation of maxillofacial surgery, and after the war, they did establish the Plastic &Maxillofacial units distributed in all the country where sited in the presence of industrial cities and near the high roads through the NHS, great understanding the disease of the TMJ occurred [2].

It was a challenge for all craniomaxillofacial surgery and research to understand the disease that affects the TMJ. In the fifties, sixties, and seventies, it was great difficulty to understand the problems and disease of the TMJ.

Ankylosis of the TMJ unpleasant disease was not common in western countries but exists in underdeveloped countries because of lack of education and poverties. The cause of this unpleasant disease is more probably due to trauma during childhood affecting the joint and might suppurative infection comes from otitis media, we studied this disease, that not only the patient cannot chew food with facial deformities and disturbance of anatomy of the upper respiratory tract and complaining from sleep apnoea [3].

In the mid seventy of last century, we did find the solution for management of people suffering from this disease by advocating two-part chrome cobalt prosthesis to restore the function of the TMJ in adults. We faced another problem, the disease once affect children not only damage the function but also the growth of the mandible and midface [3–6].

In the mid seventy, David Poswillo 1974 advocated the Costo-Chondral graft and its application for reconstruction of the damaged TMJ for restoration of growth of the condyle. It was a revolution in surgery of the TMJ at that time and he supported his work by experimental studies on Monkeys, this graft was Widley used for reconstruction of TMJ in both children and adults for 3 decades [7].

IntechOpen

In the mid eighty of last century 1986, we did advocate the Chondro-Osseous graft for reconstruction of the TMJ for restoring growth of the condyle as growth centre in children, this graft proved to be much superior to Costo-Chondral graft, because the cartilage cap in Chondro-Osseous graft is more stable and the other might dislodge during operation and also might pneumonia of the thorax have developed and unpredictable growth pattern occurred and reported [8].

We carried out an experimental study on rabbits to understand the cytology of the Chondro-Osseus graft, the articular part of the graft consisted from dense fibrocartilage layer as the first layer, the second layer consisting of several layers of round mesenchymal stem cells, the third layer consists from several immature chondrocyte and passing through series of operations to mature the chondrocyte and the fourth layer consist from bone marrow and osteoblast cells [8].

This graft proved to be an ideal graft substitute to the condyle for restoring growth, remodeling and repair of the TMJ. The graft was applied in cases of ankylosed joint in children, in hypoplasia of the condyle, and in first arch syndrome.

Fred Henny in the mid sixty suggested the use of high shave operation of the condyle to decrease the growth of the condyle in hyperplasia of the condyle during puberty, and he did use this operation for relief of pain in osteoarthritic changes of the articular layer in old people, he supported his technique by application of few drops of hydrocortisone. This technique was very popular during the sixty and seventy last century [1].

Further research done by experiment on rabbits of bone grafting has been done recently to understand the cellular changes associated with bone grafting, we did observe that the graft was invaded by capillaries after 24 hours coming from periosteum and muscles covering and mesenchymal stem cells coming from bone marrow of stump and platelets growth factor (PGF) coming from platelets, the success of bone grafting is based on decortication of both stump of bone and graft with rigid fixation [2].

2. Recent improvements in diagnosis and diagnostic tools

The improvement of diagnostic tools recently of the TMJ were greatly improved by using an electronic stethoscope for detection of disc movement and condyle relation in cases of hyper mobility of TMJ. Also, biomechanics of the TMJ studied the movements of the condyle and anatomy of muscles functions and the results were optimistic. The orthodontic treatment is required for correction of occlusion because mal occlusion creates a disturbance in relation of the disc to the condyle. Pain usually associated with TMJ disease should be eliminated from trigeminal neuralgia, migraine, muscle spasm, and tooth pain [1].

More work and research have been carried out recently by application of physiotherapy for managements of temporomandibular joint disease for the relief of pain and spasm of joint muscles.

Arthrography is an excellent diagnostic aid for studying the disease of disc displacement and deformity of the disc including disc perforation. Another diagnostic tool is the MRI for studying the soft tissue component of the TMJ including disc pathology and even perforation of the disc which might require meniscoplasty by using temporal fascia for repair of the disc or we might use sialastic sheet of 1 mm to replace the disc [1].

Recurrent dislocation and subluxation are unpleasant diseases; the patient became nervous, upset, and depressed. It affects both young and old people; the situation is that when the patient once dislocated his condyle of the joint and became unable to close his moth. Acute dislocation can be managed in the clinic by giving local anaesthesia to the joint, and the mandible was reduced by our new technique by standing behind the patient, and the operator should ask the patient to be relaxed. The surgeon hold the body of the mandible and using the angle as pivot by unilateral rotation of the condyle; the dislocated condyle jumped to glenoid fossa and other side reduced immediately. This technique been used instead by Hypo crate, 2000 BC technique by pushing the mandible downward and backward, which is no more accepted and very destructive [9].

Chronic recurrent dislocation or subluxation occurred due to lax capsule and resorption of articular eminence more common in Yamen, Somalia, Sudan, and Saudia Arabia due to habitual chewing of Qat for several hours per day; The Qat with amphetamine-like action passing through two stages. In the first, he became alert and in the second stage became fully relaxed and sleepy. Qat is a very destructive drug-like action to TMJ by converting the passive movement to active movements with severe damage to TMJ [1, 9].

The most recent technique for reconstruction of the TMJ for the above disease of chronic recurrent sub-luxation using temporal fascial of finger like with inferiorly based used for reconstruction of the lateral wall and anterior wall of laxed capsule for reinforcement and using a piece of bone graft impacted in ostectomy site in front of atrophied eminence as an obstacle for further movement of the condyle forward [9].

Author details

Raja Kummoona
Emeritus Professor of Craniomaxillofacial Surgery, Iraqi Board for Medical Specializations, Baghdad, Iraq

*Address all correspondence to: raja_kummoona@hotmail.com

References

[1] Kummoona R. History of maxillofacial surgery. In: Kummoona R, editor. Disease of the Temporomandibular Joint, Surgical Reconstruction, Clinical & Experimental Studies. New York: Science PG; 2014

[2] Kummoona R. Prologue: Foundation and Progress of craniofacial surgery. In: Al-masri, Kummoona, editors. Maxillofacial Surgery and Craniofacial Deformity, Practices and Updates. UK, London: Intech Open; 2020

[3] Kummoona R. Temporomandibular joint reconstruction with a 2-part chrome-cobalt prosthesis, Chondro-osseous graft and Sialastic: Clinical & Experimental Studies. The Journal of Craniofacial Surgery. 2009;**20**:2125-2135

[4] Hunter J. The Natural History of Human Teeth. 2nd ed. London: J Johnson; 1778

[5] Moss ML. The primary of functional matrices in orofacial growth. Dental Practioner and Dental Records. 1968;**19**(2):65-73

[6] Kummoona R. Kummoona two-part prosthesis for replacement of the temporomandibular joint. EC Orthopedic. 2020;**11**(8):01-10

[7] Poswillo DE. Surgery of the temporomandibular joint. Oral Sciences Reviews. 1974;**6**:84-118

[8] Kummoona R. Temporomandibular joint Ankylosis that affect children and reconstruction by Kummoona Chonro-Ossous graft. EC Paediatrics. 2018;**7**(11):1035-1036

[9] Kummoona R. Surgical managements of subluxation and dislocation of the temporomandibular joint: Clinical & Experimental Studies. Journal of Craniofacial Surgery. 2010;**21**(6):1692-1697

Section 2

Surgical Managements of the Temporomandibular Joint

Chapter 2

Surgical Reconstruction of the Temporomandibular Joint

Raja Kummoona

Abstract

This chapter provides a comprehensive overview of the temporomandibular joint (TMJ), including its embryonic development, anatomy, and physiology. It also discusses techniques for management and reconstruction in TMJ disorders, such as TMJ ankylosis (in children and adults), first arch syndromes, and chronic and acute TMJ dislocation and subluxation.

Keywords: temporomandibular joint (TMJ), ankylosis, dislocation, subluxation, chondro-osseous graft

1. Introduction

In 1962, Melvin Moss introduced the functional matrix theory, which proposed that the growth of the face is due to functional demand of the periosteal matrix of the facial skeleton. In 1771, John Hunter was the first to nominate the condyle as the primary growth center of the facial skeleton in his book *The Natural History of the Human Teeth* [1]. Moss's theory was more accepted for many years, but we believe the true nature of the growth of the facial skeleton lies within a combination of both theories [2].

2. Embryonic development of the TMJ

Much research has been carried out to understand the formation and development of the mandible and TMJ. The mandible develops from the first pharyngeal arch, which is formed from the neural crest that originates in the mid and hind brain of neural folds. The TMJ develops from mesenchymal condensation of cells, these cells separating between development of squamous portion of temporal bone from condylar cartilage which form the dorsal surface of developing condyle. The early movements of these cells to form the primary TMJ occur at embryonic age 4 months.

Three phases of TMJ development have been reported. The first phase is called the blastemic stage, which occurs during weeks 7–8 of embryonic development. Organization of the condyle, articular disc, and capsule begin at this stage. The second phase is the cavitation stage, during which the inferior joint cavity begins to form at embryonic age 9–11 weeks. This stage involves initial formation of the inferior joint cavity (week 9) and the start of condyle chondrogenesis (week 11). Organization of the superior joint cavity also begins in week 11. The third phase is the maturation stage (after 12 weeks of embryonic development).

The two slits of the joint cavities and the intervening disc form at 12 weeks of embryonic life and the mesenchyme around the joint forms the capsule and the synovial fluid [3].

3. Anatomy and physiology of the TMJ

The TMJ is a synovial joint, unique among all other human body joints because it is the only mobile joint of the craniomandibular part where the mandible articulates with the skull base. It is a highly specialized joint consisting of two compartments. The articular part is covered by fibrocartilage, while other joints are covered by hyaline cartilage. The jaw bones that articulate with it carry teeth and its work is synchronized on both sides like that of the eyes. The TMJ allows for more than 2000 hinge and sliding movements per day in both active masticatory and passive movements like talking, swallowing, and yawning. It is one of the most active joints in the human body.

The ligaments of the TMJ are strong and tough surrounding the condyle and glenoid fossa. There are two types: primary ligaments (temporomandibular ligaments) consisting of outer oblique and inner horizontal ligaments, and minor ligaments (styloid-mandibular and sphenoid-mandibular ligaments) that work as supportive tissue to the capsule. Other accessory ligaments define the border movements of the TMJ.

The disc or meniscus consisted from 4 parts anterior band attached to upper fibers of lateral pterygoid muscle and the lower part of the lateral pterygoid of strong muscle fibers were attached to condylar fossa. The intermediate zone is the area between the anterior and posterior bands, which are positioned normally on the head of the condyle in a closed mouth.

The posterior part of the disc is an elastic recoil fiber attached to the posterior part of the capsule. When the condyle moves forward the posterior band moves with it. Any disorganization between the two parts of the muscle fibers and failure of the posterior band to move with the condyle can cause internal derangements and clicking in the jaw.

TMJ function is controlled by a complex series of reflexes for muscular movement of mastication.

The TMJ consist of two compartments separated by the meniscus: the superior compartment and the inferior compartment. The synovial joint is located in front of the auditory meatus.

Condylar movements are unique. The condyle can move, swing, and rotate within the glenoid fossa, but its movements are limited by ligaments and surrounding muscles.

Synovial lining of the capsule form Ville in both upper and lower joint cavity to secrete fluid for lubrication and the synovial membrane provide sera-mucinous fluid for lubrication and protein for nourishment of the fibro-cartilage part of the joint.

One of the most important functions of synovial fluid that in sudden load exerted on the TMJ, lubrication occurred by squeeze film, sufficiently viscus to be squeezed slowly to persist the long enough to support the load excreted in a short time under sustained high load. The nature of lubrication was a boundary rubbing take place between the layers of large molecules absorbed in the cartilage surface and failure of lubrication causes great damages to cartilaginous part of the TMJ [3].

4. Development and growth of the TMJ

The mandible is formed and developed as a membranous bone originating from mesenchymal tissue [4].

4.1 Theories governing the growth of the facial skeleton

In his 1771 book *The Natural History of the Human Teeth*, John Hunter stated that growth of the mandible occurred as result of activation of the growth center in the condyle [1].

The functional matrix hypothesis introduced by Melvin Moss in 1962 proposed that growth of the mandible and facial skeleton occur due to functional demand of the periosteal matrix of the muscles of mastication [2].

The author believes that the true nature of the growth of the facial skeleton lies within a combination of both theories. To support his hypothesis, the author performed experiments on newly born rabbits in which he excised their condyles. After three months the rabbits showed severe deformities of their lower jaws and their mandibles were twisted to the affected side.

4.2 Functional activity of the TMJ

There are two types of movements in the TMJ: passive and active. Passive movements are used for speaking, laughing, yawning, singing, swallowing, and smoking. Active movements are used for the masticatory process, which is coordinated by four receptors.

Ruffini receptors function as static mechanoreceptors that position the mandible. Pacinian corpuscles are dynamic mechanoreceptors that accelerate movements during reflexes. The Golgi-Mazzoni corpuscles function as static mechanoreceptors for protection of themselves.

4.3 Histology of newly growing condyle

A newly growing condyle consists of four layers. The first layer is the articular fibrocartilage layer, the second layer consists of several zones of small, round mesenchymal stem cells, the third layer consists of an immature chondrocyte and newly formed osteoblasts, and the fourth layer consists of the mature trabecular bone with bone marrow in between and osteoblasts.

4.4 Reconstruction techniques for TMJ diseases

4.4.1 TMJ ankylosis in children

TMJ ankylosis is a painful disease that limits the opening of the mouth due to fusion of the condyle with the glenoid fossa in the skull base. Difficulties in mastication and swallowing are obvious signs.

There are three types of TMJ ankylosis: fibrous, bony, or a combination of both.

Facial deformity is obvious; the mandible is twisted to the affected side with short ramus and bowing of the lower border on the affected side, making a depression or concavity called the antegonial notch. This notch is a diagnostic sign of ankylosis with hyperplasia of the coronoid process. The floor of the mouth is underdeveloped and the tongue is in the retro position with changes and deformity of the upper respiratory tract, hyperplasia of epiglottis, and deformity of the larynx. The trachea is deviated and shifted to the affected side and the larynx is positioned more anterior.

These changes cause great difficulties in intubation during anesthesia by blind intubation and thus anesthesia should be done via guided endoscopic tube. With difficulties in intubation, a tracheotomy might be indicated.

The cause of this disease is mainly trauma to the chin in childhood, transmitted through the long access of the ramus to the condyle.

The condyle is a spongy type and vascular in children with short nek, the traumatic injuries to the condyle was crushing the condyle with fragmentation of the meniscus and damages to cartilaginous part of the TMJ.

Bleeding inside the joint causing hemarthrosis and the trauma may extend to the base of skull causing injuries to petrous bone and sagittal sutures of the base of skull the quelea for that was callus formation in the base of skull changing the length of transverse axis and longitudinal axis of the skull base.

Bleeding that occurs due to injuries to petrous bone of skull base, come out with CSF from the ear due to rupture of tympanic membrane. This type of case should be considered a head injury case and should be managed as such.

Surgical management of ankylosis in children is quite different from that in adults where the deformity of the facial skeleton already exists and growth is diminished.

In children, our choice is to use the Kummoona chondro-osseous graft for reconstruction of the TMJ after excision of all ankylosed bone with excision of hyper elongated coronoid process and reattachment of all muscles surrounding the ramus [5].

The chondro-osseous graft is harvested from the iliac crest. The length of the graft is between 4 and 5 cm and is covered by cup of 1-cm cartilage and small amount of muscle to work as the meniscus.

We approach the TMJ via modified incision starting from the periauricular region and going up the temporal region as a full-thickness fascio-cutaneous flap.

The dissection begins behind the temporalis muscle, from the posterior fibers of the temporalis muscle as a full-thickness Kummoona fascio-cutaneous flap and dissected down to the capsule of the joint. An L-shaped incision is made in the capsule to expose the ankylosed joint.

After decortication of both bone graft and ascending ramus, the graft is inserted via submandibular incision and fixed after positioning the head of the graft inside the glenoid fossa covered by muscle fibers from the iliac crest.

The graft is fixed firmly to the posterior side of the ramus using soft stainless-steel 0.5-mm wire in three points as rigid fixation to prevent any movement of the graft during function.

The aim of the chondro-osseous graft is to restore the growth potential of the mandible and midface with full functional activities required from the TMJ.

We ask the child to chew food after 3–4 days to obtain more growth by functional demand of the periosteal matrix, according to the functional matrix theory [2].

This technique has also been applied to treat first arch syndrome and hypoplasia of the condyle in children.

4.5 TMJ ankylosis in adults

TMJ ankylosis in adults can be managed using a two-part chrome–cobalt prosthesis developed by the author [6, 7]. This prosthesis is used in adults because growth of the face has already completed and thus there is no place for a chondro-osseous graft.

Before its application in humans, the prosthesis was used to replace the TMJ of *Macaca* monkeys in experiments carried out at the Royal College of Surgeons of England in 1975–1978.

The prosthesis was tested after animal scarified; the histology of the ramus carrying the shaft of implant was done by (H&E), a nice granulation tissue was formed and healthy fibroblasts were nicely formed and surrounding the prosthesis and the orientation of fibrous tissue fibers by the effect of masticatory process. Ground sections and microradiographs were also done to prove the biological viability of the prosthesis and proper orientation of the prosthesis shaft of the lower prosthesis. This TMJ prosthesis allows for full functional movements, including lateral excursion movements [7].

In our research, we found that a wide band of fibrous tissue was formed between the upper and lower parts of the prosthesis. This band prevented rubbing of metal ions between the parts, which can cause microthrombi to develop in the joint and induce necrosis and failure of the prosthesis [6, 7].

4.5.1 Reconstruction of hypoplasia of the condyle and first arch syndrome

Hypoplasia of the condyle in children can occur as result of intrauterine trauma to the condyle or trauma during birth or early childhood. The ideal technique for treating hypoplasia of the condyle is the chondro-osseous graft [8].

4.5.2 Management of first arch syndrome

First arch dysplasia syndrome or hemifacial microsomia is a congenital disease caused by early embryonic occlusion of the stapedial artery, the nutrient vessel of the first and second arches. There are three types of first arch deformities: mild, moderate, and severe.

The mild form is characterized by slight deformity of the ear and presence of small Tages in front of the ear with underdeveloped mandible, condyle, and masseter muscle. The condyle might be absent, but abnormal formation of bone simulating the condyle usually double with receding chin was observed.

Moderate disease is characterized by microsomia in the affected side with slight deformity of the mandible, absence of the TMJ and upper part of the ramus, deformity of the ear, and small Tages in front of the ear as remnants of Meckel's cartilage.

The severe form is characterized by wide microsomia, severe cleft in the angle of the mouth, severe deformity of the mandible, and absence of the TMJ, the upper part of the ramus, glenoid fossa, zygomatic root of the temporal bone, and the ear.

The management of these complicated cases requires expert surgical skills. The first step is to reconstruct the zygomatic root of temporal bone via bone graft harvested either from the ilium or rib. The glenoid fossa is reconstructed via cartilage graft taken from the patient's unaffected ear, followed by reconstruction of the cleft of the angle (commissuroplasty) by measuring the upper lip from midline to the angle of the mouth on the normal side. This measurement is applied on the cleft side with excision of skin access. Reconstruction begins with closure of the oral mucosa and bringing the orbicularis muscle and surrounding muscle to modules. Finally, the overlying skin is closed.

In the second step, the platysma muscle flap is mobilized a superiorly based muscle platysma flap from side of the neck to reconstruct the atrophied masseter muscle (Kummoona Platysma Muscle Flap). After a few months, the TMJ is reconstructed via chondro-osseous graft harvested from the iliac crest because the bony graft requires bulky muscle to overlap the graft for nourishment.

The chondro-osseous graft was designed for reconstruction of the TMJ during the growth period at age 4–6 years for restoration of the growth of the mandible and midface.

The graft contains mesenchymal stem cells responsible for growth, repair, and remodeling of the TMJ before reconstruction of the ear, chin reconstruction by Sialastic implant as genioplasty, bone grafting in this area might showed resorption.

The final stage of reconstruction of the first arch is to reconstruct the ear and correct occlusion via orthodontic treatment. Osteotomy or distraction techniques may be required for correction of jaw deformities [5, 9].

4.6 TMJ dislocation and recurrent subluxation

Acute dislocation of the TMJ is always associated with pain and spasm of masseter, temporalis, and internal pterygoid muscles, leading to trismus and preventing return of the condyle to the glenoid fossa [10]. It occurs when the condyles suddenly jump out of the glenoid fossa ventral to the articular eminence and become locked anterior and superior to the articular eminence. It can result from extreme opening of the mouth, for example, during extensive dental work or yawning.

Chronic dislocation typically results from untreated TMJ dislocations, and the condyle remains displaced for an extended period. It occurs less often after trauma. Both sides of the condyle slide on articular eminence ventrally to the infratemporal fossa. In chronically dislocated unreduced condyle, the capsule becomes fused and adheres to the infratemporal fascia.

Risk factors for dislocation includes weakness of the joint capsule, anatomic aberration of the joint, or injuries to associated ligaments.

Subluxation of the TMJ is an excessive abnormal excursion of the condyle secondary to flaccidity and laxity of a capsule or a condition where the condylar head moves anterior to the eminence on wide opening of the mouth. In this case, the mouth can be closed again easily but slowly.

Acute subluxation or dislocation is always associated with pain due to presence of intra-articular effusion and muscle spasm.

Chronic recurrent dislocation or subluxation is characterized by the condyle sliding over the articular eminence and catching briefly beyond the eminence before returning to the glenoid fossa.

The pathogenesis of dislocation and recurrent subluxation secondary to weakness or laxity of the capsule has been attributed to trauma or abnormal chewing habits movements. It is found more frequently in people with general joint laxity (Ehlers-Danlos syndrome, Marfan syndrome, and juvenile rheumatoid arthritis), in older persons with laxity of ligaments, weak muscles, and bone resorption, and individuals with internal derangements of the TMJ or with occlusal disturbance. Other predisposing factors include prolonged opening of the mouth during dental treatment/ examination or during general anesthesia or bronchoscopy.

In countries like Yemen, Sudan, Somalia, and South Arabia, some TMJ disorders can be attributed to khat chewing. Khat is a plant found in Southern Arabia and East Africa known for its stimulant effects. Khat chewing is a social tradition. Daily chewing of khat produces an excessive load on the TMJ, changing its normal excursive hinge masticatory movements to habitual rotatory movement, leading to osteoarthritic changes including atrophy of the articular eminence, shallow glenoid fossa, and lax capsule and ligaments of the TMJ. The instability of the lower jaw during speech is due to the effect of khat on the brain stem. The plant exhibits amphetamine-like action and users become very talkative under its influence.

4.6.1 Management of TMJ dislocation

There are many methods for reducing dislocation of the TMJ, the most common of which is the Hippocratic method. This method involves the practitioner standing in front of the patient and placing a gloved thumb on the posterior lower molars bilaterally with fingers wrapped laterally around the mandible. Then, the practitioner pushes the jaw downward and backward to ease it back into the glenoid fossa.

Other techniques involve injecting sclerosing agents into the capsule or using autologous blood. These methods are mostly no longer used because they can cause damage to some vital structures of the joint and pain during the procedure and postoperatively.

We propose a new technique, in which the practitioner grips the patient's lower jaw from behind and using the angle of lower jaw as pivot with slight rotation on one side immediately the condyle return to its normal position in the glenoid fossa, and immediate return of the condyle in other sides to glenoid fossa. The angle of the jaw mobilizes as a pivot by rotating the mandible in one side, immediately the side reduced and followed by other side [10, 11].

4.6.2 Management of TMJ subluxation

The ideal surgical technique advocated by the author for treating chronic recurrent subluxation and dislocation involves reinforcing and supporting the weak lax capsule with an inferiorly based, finger-shaped temporal fascia flap for reconstruction of the lateral and anterior walls of the capsule.

With reconstruction of the zygomatic root of temporal bone just in front of the articular eminence by creating an ostectomy in 45 degrees towards the joint and impacted a piece of bone from iliac crest of about 1.5 cm length and 1 cm width, it works as an obstacle for forward movement of the condyle [9, 10].

4.7 TMJ osteoarthritis

Osteoarthritis is a degenerative disease of aging that causes more severe symptoms in weight-bearing joints like the ankles and hips. It usually affects the TMJ in the early stages before it spreads to other joints of the body. TMJ osteoarthritis is characterized by a breakdown of the articular fibrocartilage layer with architectural changes in the associated bone and damage and degeneration of synovial tissue causing pain in the joint.

X-ray examination of the TMJ shows osteophytes, lipping, and cyst-like lesions (Ely's cysts) with flatting of the articular layer. In the later stages, X-ray may reveal erosion of the condyle articular surface.

In advanced disease, the articular cartilage becomes less elastic with erosion of the surface of the condyle associated with vertical cleft or crack in the subchondral bone.

Reparative attempts of the joint at the periphery of the cartilage result in formation of osteophytes, lipping, and changes in the surface contour of the articular surface [3].

4.7.1 Management of TMJ osteoarthritis

In mild cases with pain and difficulty of mastication, my colleagues and I administer the intra-articular steroid methylprednisolone (injection of 80 mg 2 ml) to the superior and inferior compartments of the joint. We repeat this technique three times at two-week intervals.

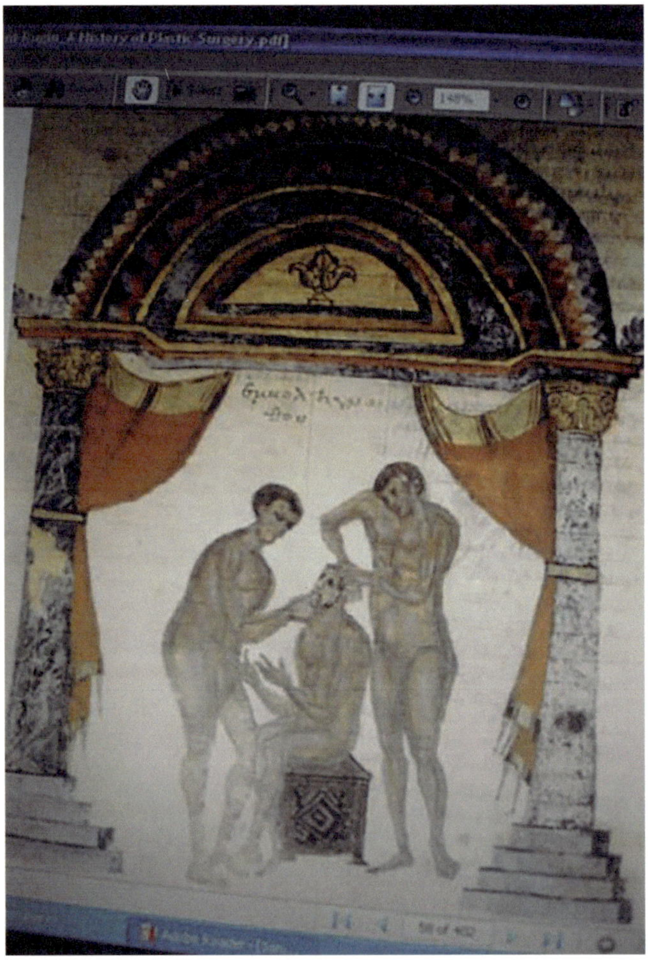

Figure 1.
Hippocratic technique for reducing dislocated condyles.

In severe cases, surgical exploration of the TMJ is applied by full thickness fascio-cutaneous flap from the periauricular area with an extension to temporal region as? Flap. An L-shaped incision is made in the capsule to expose the condyle.

Irregularities of the condyle are removed by a pear-shaped surgical bur for removing the abnormal osteophyte, lavage of the joint, and inserting a sialastic implant shaped like the meniscus to prevent any friction between the glenoid fossa and the condyle.

4.8 TMJ dysfunction

TMJ dysfunction involving clicking of the jaw with or without pain is more prevalent in women than men. Jaw clicking is due to lack of coordination between movement of the disc and head of the condyle caused by hyperactivity of strong lower muscle fibers of the lateral pterygoid muscle with upper fine muscle fibers that attach to the anterior part of the disc. Other causes include irregularities in teeth position and occlusion disturbance. In severe cases, it may be associated with muscle spasm, which can limit mouth opening, deviate the jaw, and cause pain.

Radiological examination can be conducted via arthrography by injecting radiopaque material into the lower compartment of the TMJ to demonstrate reversible or irreversible disc movement and displacement of the disc or inferior-medial movement

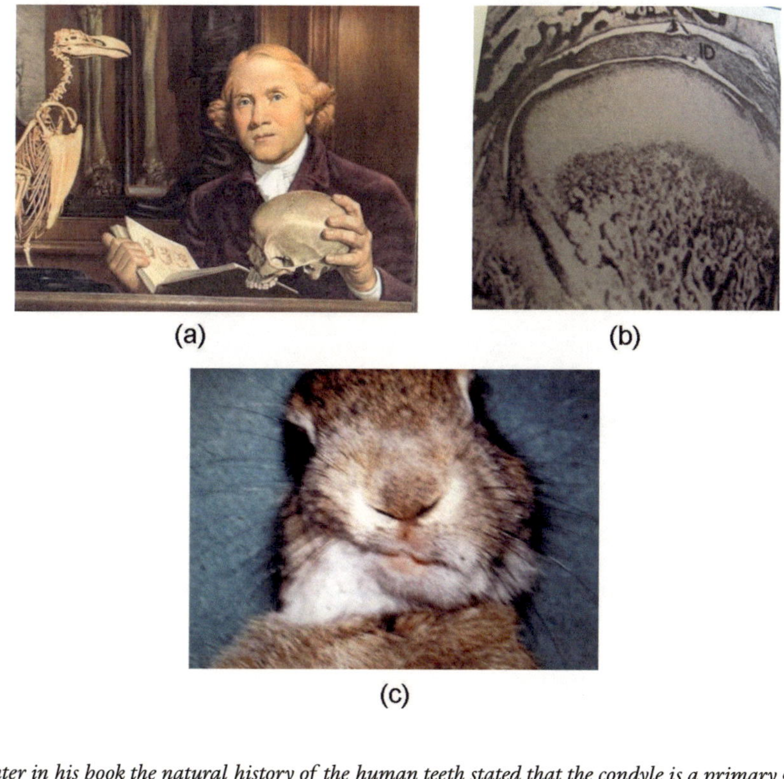

Figure 2.
a. John Hunter in his book the natural history of the human teeth stated that the condyle is a primary growth center. b. section of a newborn's condyle showing active mesenchymal stem cells. c. newly born rabbit with jaw and facial deformity three months later due to excision of condyle and prove to be a growth center.

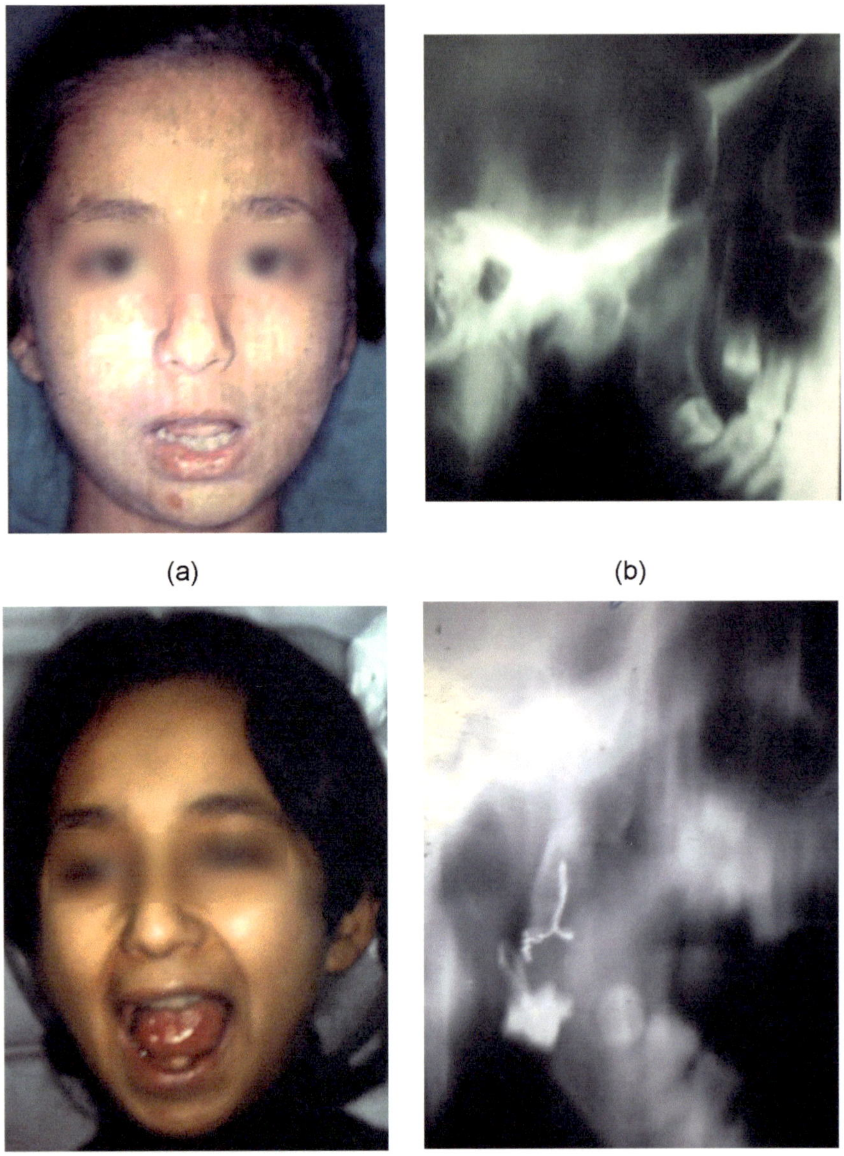

(a) (b)

(c) (d)

Figure 3.
a. A five-year-old female with ankylosis of the left TMJ. b. tomography of the left ankylosed TMJ. c. one year after reconstruction of the TMJ by chondro-osseous graft restoring normal face and normal mouth opening. d. tomography of the TMJ showing normal condyle movement created by chondro-osseous graft.

of the meniscus. Injection of radiopaque material to lower compartment of the TMJ can demonstrate disc perforation.

MRI has also been used to study changes in the head of the condyle and disc movement; however, MR is used mainly for viewing soft tissue of the TMJ.

Management of early cases of TMJ dysfunction with jaw clicking involves construction of a bite raising appliance to raise the bite or mouth opening between 2 and 3 mm to obtain proper relation between the head of the condyle and the disc where the posterior band of the disc cited on the top of the condyle. The patient should wear the bite

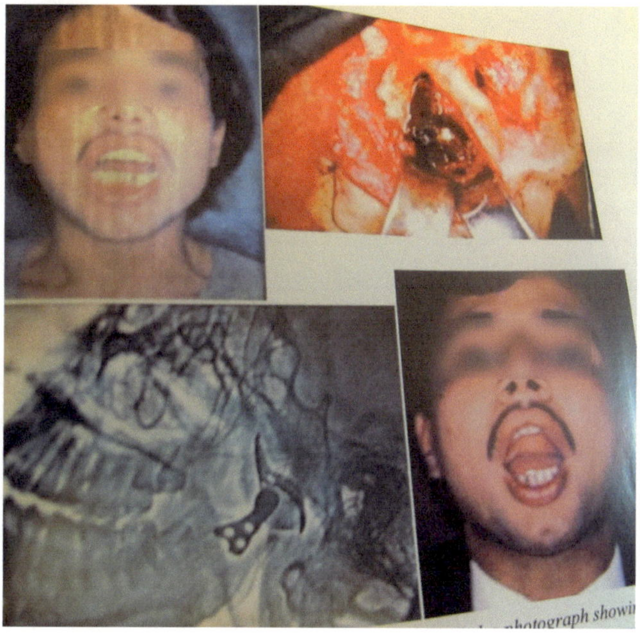

Figure 4.
Composite of four photos showing an 18-year-old man with ankylosed TMJ. First photo is preoperative and shows limited mouth opening. Second photo shows Kummoona two-part prosthesis replacing the TMJ. Third photo shows xerography X-ray of the jaw demonstrating the two-part prosthesis replacing the TMJ. Fourth photo shows the patient after 10 years with normal mouth opening.

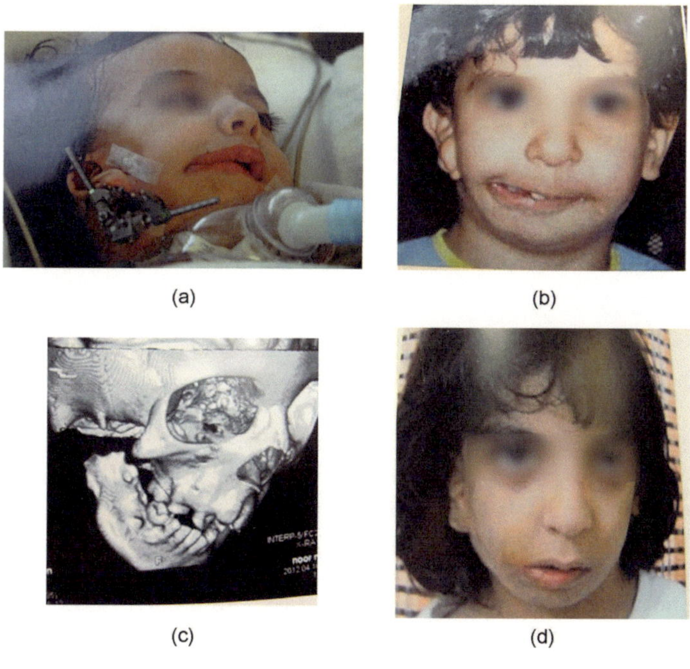

Figure 5.
a. Baby born with first arch syndrome treated with distraction techniques with poor results. b. photo showing same child at age 4 years. c. CT scan of female child showing missing ramus and zygomatic arch of temporal bone. d. two-year postoperative photo after series of operations.

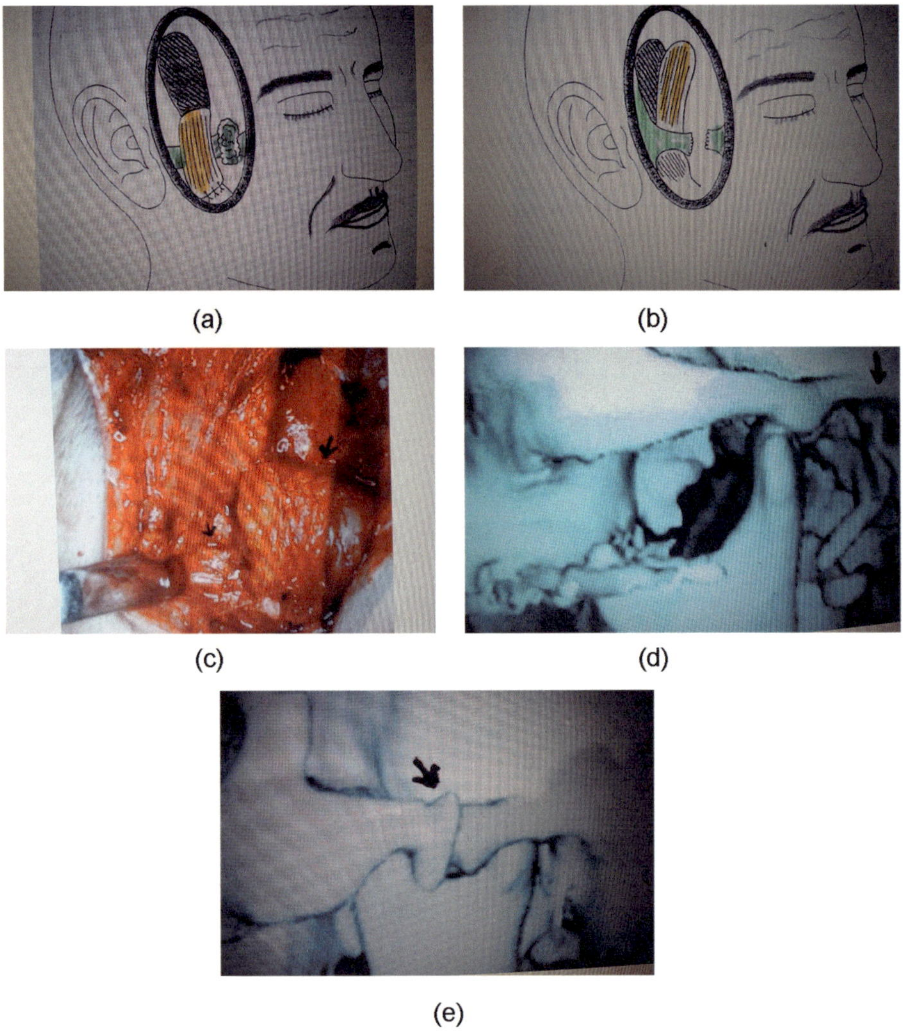

Figure 6.
a. A diagram showing design of Kummoona fascial temporal flap inferiorly based for reconstruction of lateral and anterior walls of the capsule of TMJ and site of ostectomy anterior to articular eminence of the joint. b. diagram showing temporal fascial flap rotated and used for reconstruction of the capsule and bone graft impacted in the site of ostectomy. c. photo showing temporal fascial flap mobilized to reconstruct the capsule. d. CT scan showing dislocation of the condyle. e. CT scan showing bone graft anterior to articular eminence and working as obstacle for forward movement of the condyle.

raising appliance at night. The night bite appliance was very unsuccessful method for management of TMJ dysfunction. Correction of occlusion by orthodontic treatment should be done before construction of the bite raising appliance or at the same time.

The patient should be advised not to chew hard food or gum, to avoid yawning, and not to open their mouth more than.

We prescribe an anti-inflammatory medication and muscle relaxant to relieve muscle spasm and pain in the joint for one week.

Botulinum toxin A (Botox-A) has been used to relieve the hyperactivity of lower fibers of the lateral pterygoid muscle. It has shown some efficacy in clinical studies involving female patients. We do not recommend blood injection to the joint because it can cause damage to the cartilaginous part of the TMJ (**Figures 1–7**).

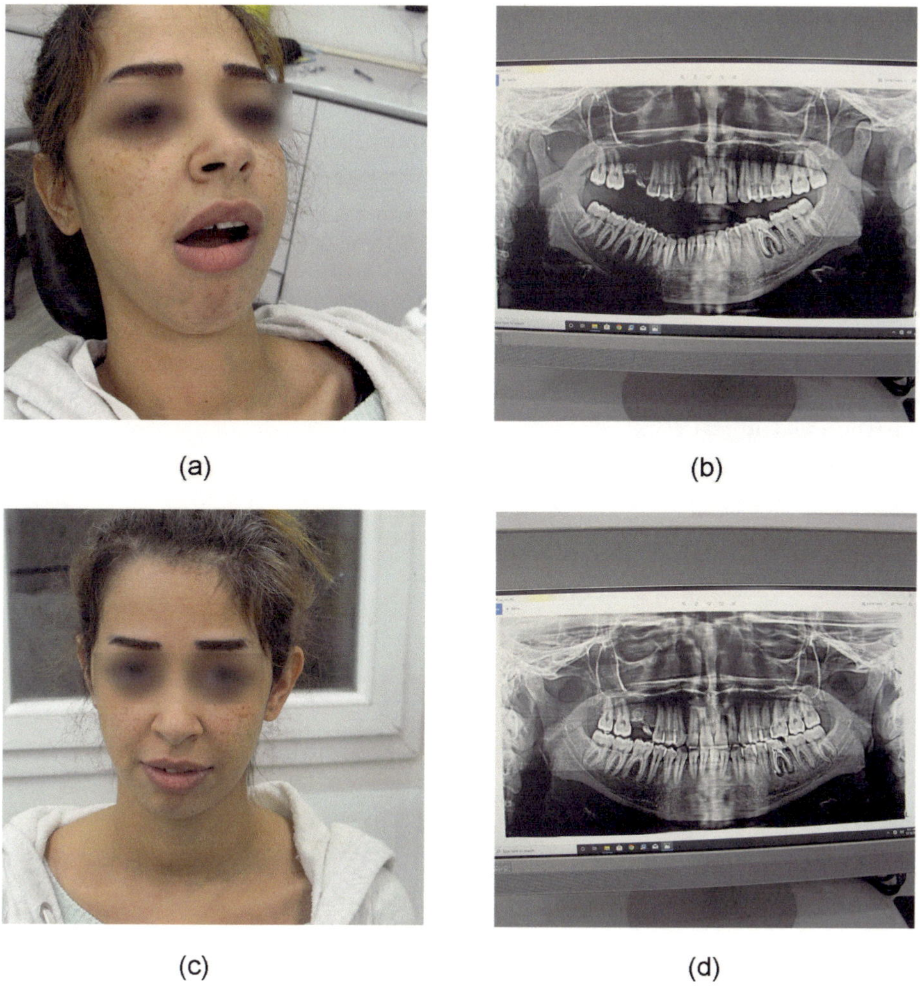

Figure 7.
a. Young woman with acute dislocation of the condyle. b. X-ray OPG showing dislocation of the condyle. c. photograph showing normal face after immediate reduction of dislocated condyle by Kummoona manual technique. d. X-ray OPG showing the condyle in the glenoid fossa after reduction.

Author details

Raja Kummoona
Craniomaxillofacial Surgery, Iraqi Board for Medical Specializations, Baghdad, Iraq

*Address all correspondence to: raja_kummoona@hotmail.com

References

[1] Hunter J. The Natural History of Human Teeth. 2nd ed. London: J Johnson; 1778

[2] Moss ML. The primary of functional matrices in orofacial growth. Dental Practioner and Dental Records. 1968;**19**(2):65-73

[3] Kummoona R. Disease of the temporomandibular joint, surgical reconstruction, Clinical &Experimental Studies. Book, ed, Raja Kummoona. New York: Science Publication group; 2014

[4] Poswillo DE. Surgery of the temporomandibular joint. Oral Sciences Reviews. 1974;**6**:84-118

[5] Kummoona R. Temporomandibular joint Ankylosis that affect children and reconstruction by Kummoona Chondro-Osseous1 graft. EC Pediatrics. 2018;**7**(11):1035-1036

[6] Kummoona R. Temporomandibular joint reconstruction with a 2-part chrome-cobalt prosthesis, chondro-osseous graft and Sialastic: Clinical and experimental studies. The Journal of Craniofacial Surgery. 2009;**20**:2125-2135

[7] Kummoona R. Kummoona two part prosthesis for replacement of the temporomandibular joint. EC Orthopedic. 2020;**11**(8):01-10

[8] Kummoona R. Temporomandibular joint reconstruction by Kummoona techniques. EC Orthopedics. 2022;**13**(3):07-08

[9] Kummoona R. Dislocation and subluxation of the temporomandibular joint. EC Pediatrics. 2020;**S1**(03):13-15

[10] Kummoona R. Managements of subluxation and dislocation of the temporomandibular joint: Clinical and experimental studies. Journal of Craniofacial Surgery. 2010;**21**(6):1692-1697

[11] Kummoona R. Surgical reconstruction of the temporomandibular joint for chronic subluxation and dislocation. Journal of Oral and Maxillofacial Surgery. 2001;**30**:344-348

Chapter 3

Orthognatic Surgery With Reconstruction of the Temporomandibular Joint

Vladimír Machoň and Michal Beňo

Abstract

Orthognathic surgery with reconstruction of the temporomandibular joint (TMJ) addresses conditions where dentofacial deformity (DFD) is present along with damage to the temporomandibular joint. A stable TMJ without signs of pathology is a basic prerequisite for successful orthognathic surgery. If pathology is present, it is necessary to first address the condition of the TMJ (through conservative, mini-invasive and surgical methods). Only after the condition of the TMJ is stabilized is it possible to surgically address DFD. Orthognathic surgery in conjunction with TJR is performed in a single operation, where precise planning of these surgical procedures is vital for their successful execution.

Keywords: temporomandibular joint, orthognatic surgery, TMJ replacement, total joint prosthesis, dentofacial deformity, temporomandibular disorders

1. Introduction

Orthognathic surgery with reconstruction of the temporomandibular joint (TMJ) addresses conditions where dentofacial deformity (DFD) is present along with damage to the temporomandibular joint. Basically, these are conditions where [1, 2]:

1. DFD is the result of condylar pathology

2. there is primarily DFD, but with developing TMD.

The aim of treating these conditions is:

1. to achieve good facial esthetics and satisfactory occlusion, airway and breathing capabilities

2. to reduce or eliminate pain and restore full functionality of the temporomandibular joint

This goal is achieved through standard orthognathic surgical techniques (sagittal osteotomy, LeFort I osteotomy, genioplasty), together with the use of TMJ

IntechOpen

reconstruction techniques in a single surgical procedure. Patients may also choose two-stage surgery (TMJ reconstruction and subsequent orthognathic surgery), however performing both procedures in a single operation reduces the impact of general anesthesia, reduces the overall duration of surgery and the patient need only recover once, which is an indisputable benefit. Nonetheless, performing both procedures at the same time requires flawless preparation and planning [3–7].

In general, a stable TMJ is required for a stable orthognathic outcome. If the TMJ is pathologically altered, then correcting facial asymmetry while ignoring the pathological condition of the TMJ can lead to a recurrence of facial asymmetry, malocclusion, and exacerbation of joint problems [1].

2. TMJ indication for joint reconstruction

Patients with TMJ pathology and concomitant DFD may show typical TMJ symptoms (limited jaw movement, presence of TMJ pain, occlusal disturbance). Nevertheless, a second group of patients exhibit clinically asymptomatic TMJ, where the impact on DFD is only revealed by imaging methods [1, 3]. In these patients, the condition of the TMJ represents a potential risk to the long-term stability of the outcome of orthognathic surgery in the event of progressing TMJ pathology. The question is whether to choose preventive TMJ reconstruction in these patients or to address the condition of the joint by other methods [3]. This problem is especially evident in the diagnosis of idiopathic condylar resorption (ICR), where some authors prefer stabilizing the joint (bite guards, drug therapy, TMJ open surgery) or performing preventive TMJ reconstruction [8–10].

2.1 Indications for joint reconstruction during orthognathic surgery include

1. conditions where joint function is limited due to a change in condylar quality (severe osteoarthritis, end-stage internal derangement, severe septic TMJ arthritis, avascular necrosis, systemic connective tissue and autoimmune diseases, synovial chondromatosis, primary condylar tumors such as osteoma, osteochondroma, diffuse tenosynovial giant cell tumor)

2. reduced condyle height due to pathological TMJ processes (idiopathic condylar resorption, inflammatory arthritis, severe osteoarthritis, severe septic TMJ arthritis, systemic connective tissue and autoimmune diseases)

3. absence of the condyle (congenital and developmental defects affecting TMJ structures, conditions after condylar resection for traumatic impairment or resection of TMJ tumors)

4. TMJ ankylosis

5. conditions following previous unsatisfactory surgeries

A clear contraindication for TMJ reconstruction to address DFD (and in general) are patients with disco-condylar complex disorders (clinically manifested by acoustic phenomena, locking, limited jaw movement) and patients with chronic pain who have no obvious joint pathology (e.g., myofascial pain) [2].

3. Options for TMJ reconstruction in patients with dentofacial deformities

TMJ reconstruction can generally be achieved by using two basic methods:

1. Use of autogenous materials (costochondral graft, sternoclavicular graft, fibular graft, chondro-osseous graft harvested from iliac crest)

2. Use of allogeneic materials (where the most common materials are titanium, a cobalt chromium alloy and polyethylene)

Autogenous materials are popular for TMJ reconstruction in pediatric patients (especially costochondral graft) due to their growth capacity. However, the unpredictability of growth is a problem (excessive growth or no growth), as well as unpredictable bone graft stability and donor site morbidity. The use of allogenous materials is not suitable for TMJ reconstruction with concurrent orthognathic surgery [11–13].

Allogeneic prostheses can be partial or total.

Partial replacement (typically a prosthetic replacement of the mandibular condyle, which is inserted into the joint fossa) is again not a suitable for DFD. The long-term use of these prostheses is associated with an increased risk of fossa resorption due to direct contact of the head of the prosthesis with the bone fossa [13].

The ideal solution for TMJ reconstruction with DFD is total joint replacement (TJR).

Total joint replacement consists of [14, 15]:

1. fossa replacement (the prosthesis is manufactured from UHMWPE - ultra-high molecular weight polyethylene)

2. condylar replacement. The actual head of the prosthesis is made of chromium-cobalt alloy and the fixative part of the prosthesis is made of titanium. Chromium-cobalt alloy has the ability to bind with titanium, it is strong, with a highly polishable and biocompatible surface. It has excellent properties like the surface of the head of the physiological joint in relation to the polyethylene fossa and represents the orthopedic standard for total TMJ endoprostheses.

Total prostheses are available in two versions- stock prostheses and patient-fitted prostheses [15, 16].

Stock prostheses are usually manufactured in several sizes, with the ideal size of prosthesis components selected during surgery [16]. If these prostheses are used in orthognathic surgery, it must be kept in mind that this is an altogether compromise solution. Stock prostheses have the same shape and mandibular advancement is usually only achieved as a result of the inappropriate distal inclination of the prosthesis, or by moving the prosthesis behind the posterior branch of the mandible. An ideal result can only be achieved by using patient-fitted prostheses, whose shape is designed to concurrently allow the planned repositioning of the lower jaw (**Figure 1**). Another advantage of patient-fitted prostheses is their improved fit and osseointegration, thus resulting in less friction and micromovement, better stability and potentially longer mean durability [17, 18]. When the zygomatic arch and glenoid fossa were absent, the

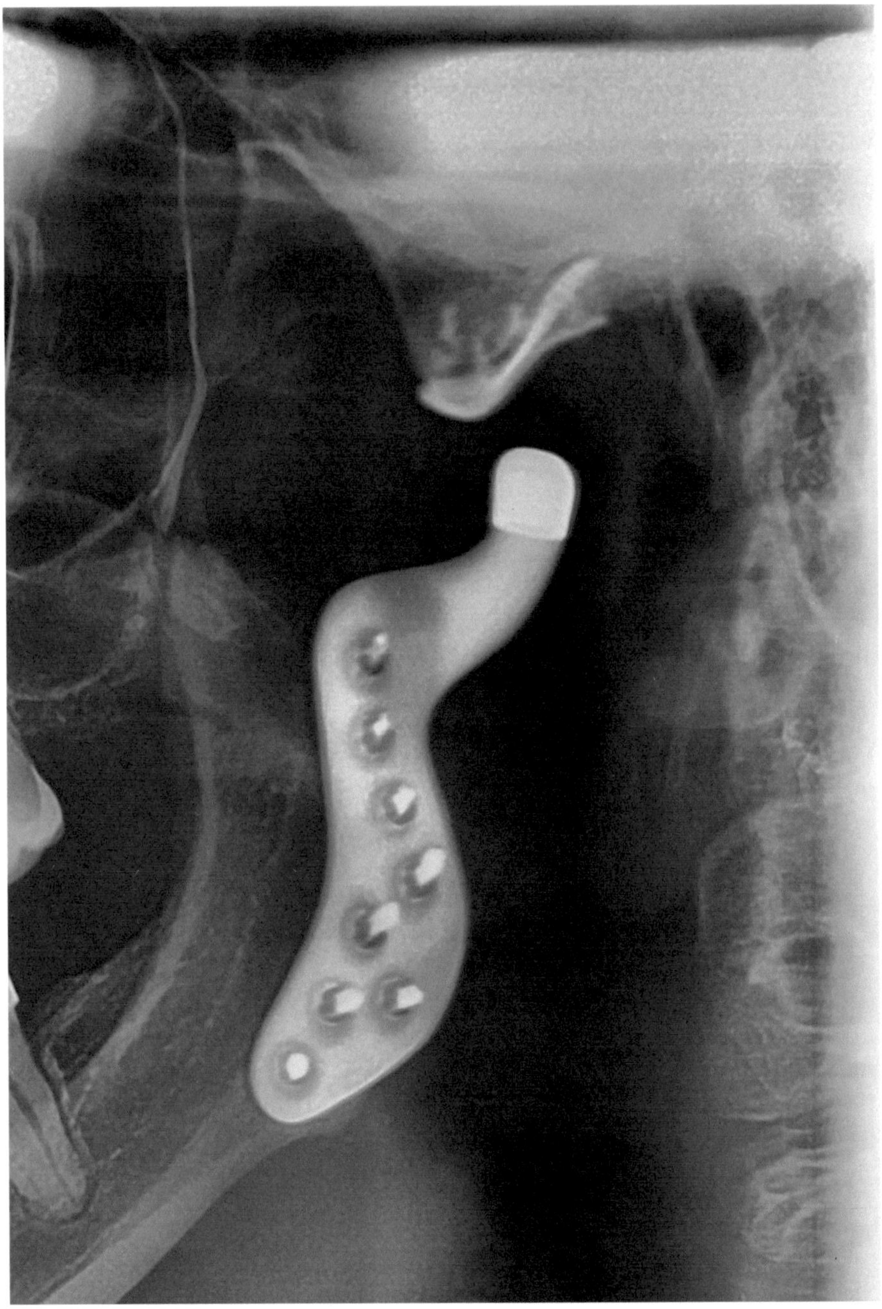

Figure 1.
TMJ prosthesis design enabling mandibular advancement.

fossa component was custom-fitted to the base of the skull and lateral temporal bone morphology [11] (**Figures 2** and **3**).

Relative contraindications of alloplastic total TMJ replacement are [19, 20]:

1. uncontrolled systemic disease

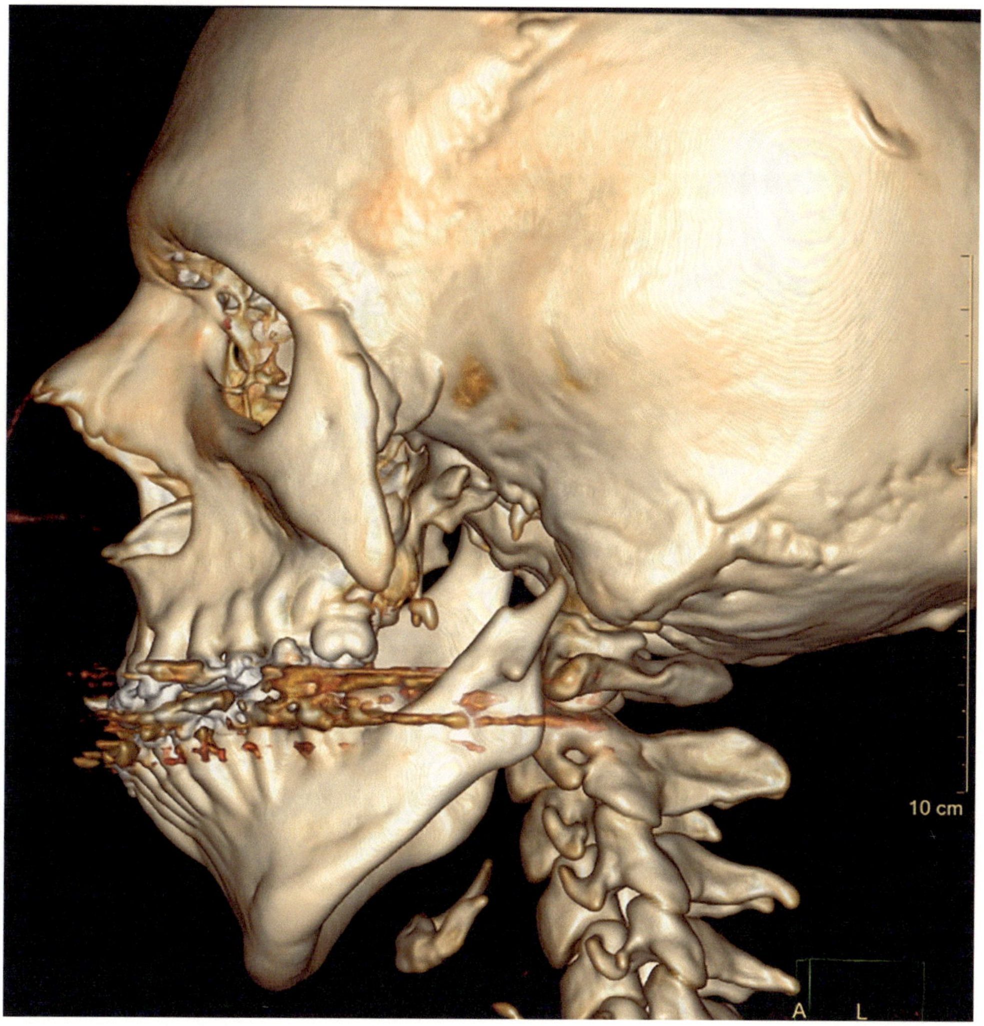

Figure 2.
22 years old man with HFM (absence of joint structures and absence of zygomatic arch).

2. active infection at the surgical site

3. allergy to the implant/prosthesis material.

Today, the previously unequivocal refusal to use TJR in pediatric patients with a growing skeleton [14] is changing, as it is no longer considered an unsuitable indication [21, 22]. Growth activity of the mandible is observed when employing TJR even in growing skeletons [21]. The use of TJR of the TMJ in children is possible in the following indications [21]:

1. High inflammatory TMJ arthritis unresponsive to other modalities of treatment

2. Recurrent fibrosis and/or bony ankylosis unresponsive to other modalities of treatment

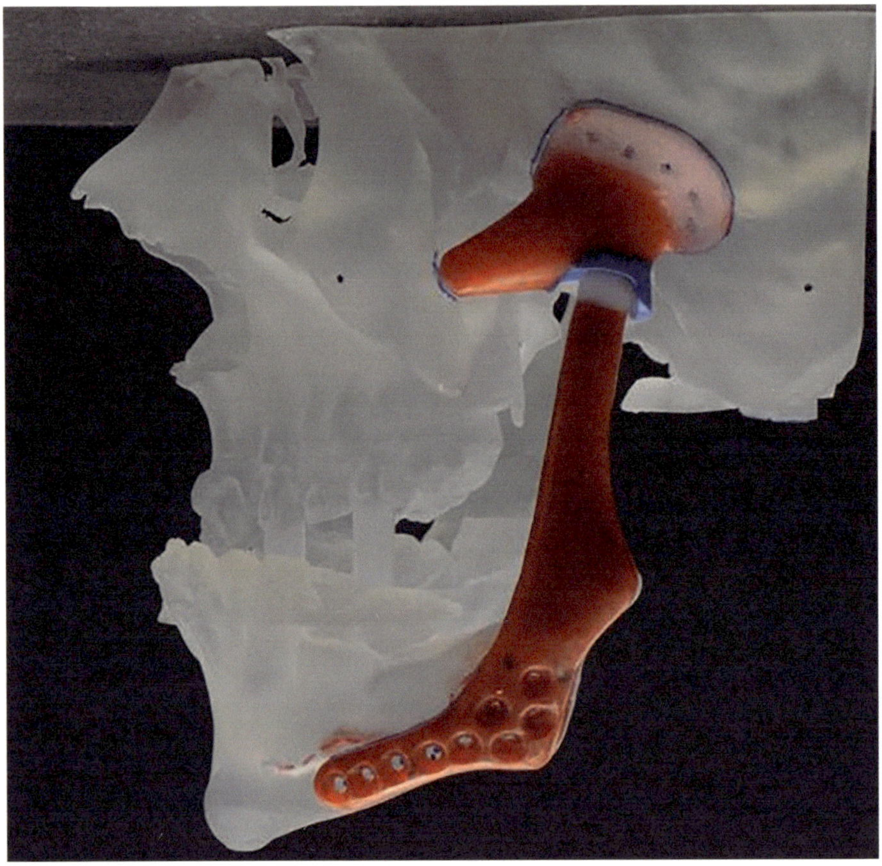

Figure 3.
22 years old man with HFM (planned reconstruction of joints structures and zygomatic arch).

3. Failed tissue grafts (bone and soft tissue)

4. Loss of vertical mandibular height and/or occlusal relationship because of bony resorption, trauma, developmental abnormalities, or pathological lesions.

It must be realized that TJR is joint replacement that is not equivalent to the physiological joint. TJR does not allow the same movement as the physiological joint. The components of the prosthesis mainly allow rotational movement, while the physiological joint allows rotation, as well as translational movement. Joint replacements only exhibit slight translation (pseudo-translation), which causes deviations in mouth opening in unilateral TJR (movement deviates to the side of the TJR). Some authors report improved translational movement when performing lateral pterygoid muscle reattachment [23, 24].

4. Orthodontic preparation of the patient

The initial consultation between the doctor and patient is important for successful treatment. The purpose of the consultation is to consider the options of surgical treatment, but also to acquaint the patient with the limits and complications of treatment.

The patient is acquainted with the reasons why TMJ reconstruction is planned. It is important to know the patient's expectations and the reasons why they decided to address their DFD. Of course, it is essential to temper any unrealistic expectations the patient may have (both in terms of correcting the DFD and eliminating TMJ problems).

An initial consultation at the authors' workplace is always held in the presence of orthodontist, orthognathic surgeon and TMJ surgeon. Orthodontic-surgical treatment of maxillary anomalies is a team effort, in which the specific approach in all phases is the result of joint decision-making and mutual consultation by individual experts.

Only after the patient has fully understood and consented to the procedure does planning the surgery begin.

The initial interview includes photo documentation of the patient, an X-ray and cone beam CT. Stone models of the upper and lower dental arch are also required to assess occlusal conditions.

In principle, the same rules apply for orthodontic preparation as when preparing patients for orthognathic surgery. Orthodontic pre-treatment is performed using fixed devices on the upper and lower arches. The main goals of orthodontic preoperative treatment are: decompensation of the defect and the creation of regular dental arches without the constriction, and rotation of the front teeth. Postoperative intercuspidation should create conditions for a stable overbite of the incisors, i.e., a suitable incisal overjet and bite depth, with normoocclusion of the canines. For lateral teeth, intercuspidation without a crossbite should be achieved postoperatively. The width of the dental arches must be proportional to each other, the shape of the arches must allow good postoperative intercuspidation [25].

In case of transverse narrowing of the upper jaw, orthodontic preparation includes expansion of the upper jaw depending on the patient's age, i.e., ossification of the *sutura palatina* (non-surgically in growing patients with a Hyrax palatal expander, or surgically in adult patients using the SARME method - surgically assisted rapid maxillary expansion).

If the patient has a biplanar occlusal plane of the upper jaw, it is important to maintain this and prepare the patient segmentally. Segments are typically formed by osteotomy between the Central incisors into segments 17–11 and 21–27 or between the lateral incisors and canines, whereby the dental arch is divided into three segments second molar to canine, incisors, canine to second molar [26–28].

In patients with congenital defects (e.g., hemifacial microsomia) or in patients who developed ankylosis in childhood, there is often severe hypoplasia of the affected branch and body of the lower jaw. In these cases, it is appropriate to use distraction osteogenesis to extend the ramus and body of the lower jaw. This technique has the advantages of providing superior amount of bone lengthening and allows simultaneos expansion of surrounding soft tissues. This elongated bone will then facilitate the movement of the jaw to the appropriate position, significantly improving the resulting esthetic effect.

Preoperative preparation includes the removal of retained teeth and introduction of dental implants. Knowledge of the patient's general condition is also required to prepare the patient for a procedure that takes several hours. Similarly, it is important to monitor levels of vitamin D and provide supplements, where necessary (low levels are associated with the risk of impaired healing of bone fragments).

The purpose of orthodontic preparation is to create ideal dental arches suitable for stable occlusion after repositioning one or both jaws. The length of orthodontic preparation depends on how complicated the condition of the dental arches is [29–31].

Depending on the condition of the dental arches, it is possible to prepare a patient for surgery in 4 ways [30]:

1. Surgery first: this approach proceeds with orthognathic surgery without preoperative orthodontic preparation and is followed by regular postoperative dental alignment.

2. Surgery early: the patient's wish for an immediate esthetic change. In this treatment concept, the presence of severe crowding in need of extractions and complex 3D dental compensations due to facial asymmetry, including dental midline deviation, requires at least partial orthodontic preparation. As soon as severe crowding has been managed with extractions and a good amount of the required space closure is achieved, surgery is performed. In the case of severe 3D compensations and/or dental midline deviations, surgery proceeds once transverse compensations are resolved.

3. Surgery late: corresponds to the conventional approach for orthognathic surgery, i.e., the traditional sequence of preoperative orthodontics, surgery, and postoperative orthodontics.

4. Surgery only: Conceptually, a 'surgery only' protocol proceeds directly with surgery, without any previous or subsequent orthodontic treatment.

4.1 Planning orthognathic surgery

The actual planning of orthognathic surgery only begins after the completion of orthodontic preparation, when passive arches are deployed with orthodontic appliances. Planning consists of virtual surgical planning (VSP). The same CT is used for VSP as for planning joint replacement. A 3D virtual patient model is generated using a 3D planning program. This requires the aforementioned CT, as well as intraoral scans of dental arches, 3D photos and a clinical analysis of the patient. This virtual model then makes it possible to plan individual osteotomies and jaw repositioning [29, 32].

Clinical analysis of the patient involves a comprehensive examination of the patient's face before surgery. Exact measurements are made (with special attention given to the Central position of the Chin) of the mutual relationship of the lips when relaxed, the bilateral symmetry of the mandible angles, symmetry of the contour of the lower jaw line, symmetry of Chin contours and possible deviations in the soft tissues of the face. Also noted are the movement of the lips when smiling, the exposure of incisors and a possible gummy smile, the relationship and position of the dental center of the upper and lower dental arch to the center of the face, the inclination of the occlusal plane and a comparison of its inclination to the bipupillary plane [26, 33].

The virtual 3D model not only makes it possible to assess the bone structure of the facial skeleton, but also creates an image of soft tissues, which is important to get an idea of esthetic outcome and facial changes in a patient with DFD [32]. The use of modern planning technologies brings better and more predictable results [33].

The resulting position of the upper and lower jaws will enable the virtual production of surgical splints, which will be printed on a 3D printer before the surgery and will allow the jaws to be moved to the planned position during the procedure [29].

Note: An intraoral scan is clearly preferred for a scan of the dental arches rather than scanning the dental arches from the model. An intraoral scan eliminates minor deviations in the impression and plaster model.

4.2 Planning and preparation of the TMJ prosthesis

As mentioned above, patient-fitted prostheses are always used for orthognathic surgery with TJR. These are prepared and produced in the following manner [15]:

1. CT scan protocol (from the middle of the forehead to the hyoid, dorsally to the anterior edge of the foramen magnum, in 0.5–0.75 mm sections, without head support - gantry tilt 0 degrees,)

2. Occlusion scan of the upper and lower dental arches

3. Orthognathic planning, preparation of a virtual splint

4. Submission of the CT, occlusion scan and virtual splint to the company producing the prosthesis

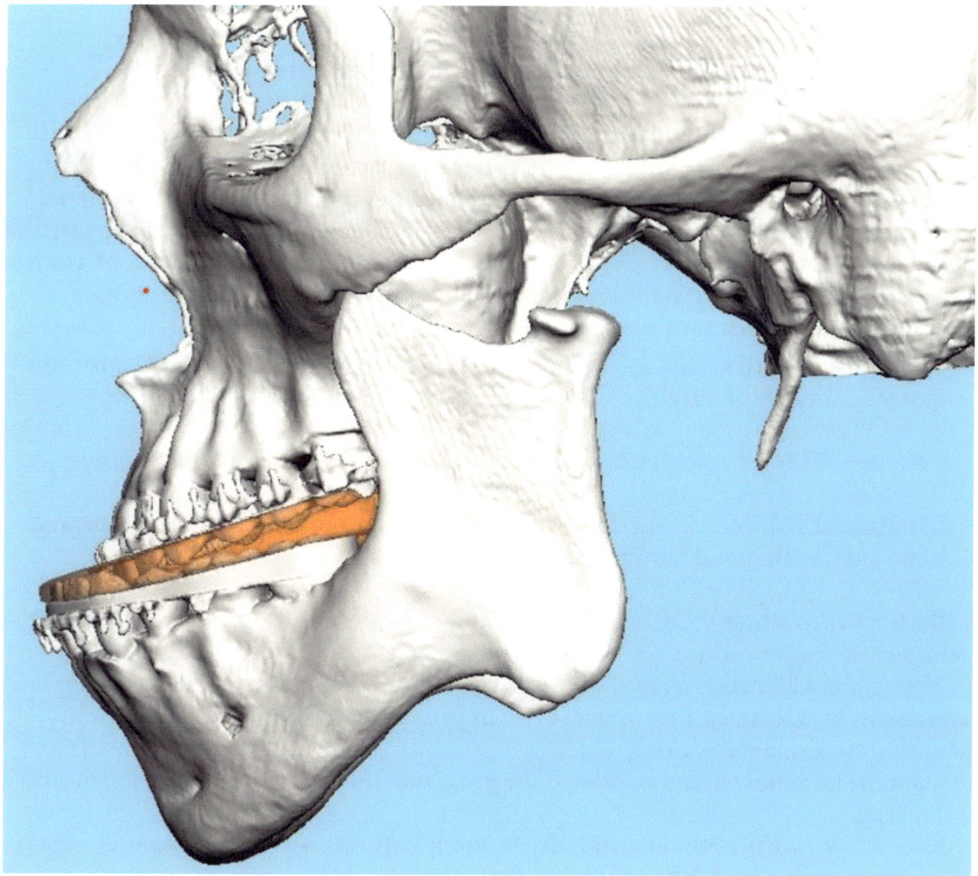

Figure 4.
CT model with final position of lower jaw and contact of coronoid process with posterior part of maxila.

5. Virtual inspection of the placement of the splint, occlusion, comparison of the resulting position of the lower jaw with the lower jaw position during orthognathic planning

6. Planning resection lines, possible modifications around the socket and mandibular branch

7. Creation of a joint replacement model

After all steps have been approved, production of the prosthesis commences.

The entire process of creating a prosthesis takes several weeks to months.

Note 1: when planning mandibular advancement, it is important to realize the differences between sagittal osteotomy advancement and total replacement advancement. During sagittal osteotomy, the position of the distal fragment (part of the branch of the mandible with the muscular and articular process) remains in the same place. In contrast, in mandibular advancement with total joint replacement, the branch is completely shifted anteriorly. This shift can cause the coronoid process to come into contact with the posterior wall of the maxila (**Figure 4**), which will in turn result in reduced jaw mobility. This is resolved through a planned coronoidectomy.

5. Algorithm for performing orthognathic surgery and TJR

It is important to remember that the surgical procedure combines both an intraoral and extraoral approach. The reconstruction of the temporomandibular joint uses extraoral approaches only, while orthognathic surgery is performed from an intraoral approach only. Due to the risk of infectious contamination of the prosthesis [2, 15, 20], it is vital to maintain strict separation of both approaches and, of course, use separate sets of instruments for both parts of the surgery. The authors also recommend separate sets of covering for the surgical field and thoroughly covering surgical wounds with sterile foils after completing individual steps of the procedure.

Basically, 2 types of surgical procedures are performed:

1. Bilateral TMJ reconstruction, with possible subsequent maxillary surgery

2. Unilateral TMJ reconstruction, split sagittal osteotomy (SSO) on the contralateral side, with possible subsequent maxillary surgery

Both types of surgery can be supplemented by intraorally performed genioplasty at the end of the procedure.

Note 1: If the fixative part of the condylar component of the prosthesis is longer and extends to at least the first molar (often in patients with hemifacial microsomia), the authors recommend waiting to perform genioplasty. This is to limit the contact between the intraoral environment and the prosthesis due to tissue preparation during genioplasty.

Note 2: Successful orthognathic surgery with TMJ reconstruction requires experience in performing both types of surgical procedures. At the authors' workplace, these procedures are performed by 2 surgeons, an orthognathic surgeon and a TMJ surgeon, at the same time.

5.1 Bilateral TMJ reconstruction, with possible subsequent maxillary surgery

1. Endaural incision for exposure of the TMJ fossa and retromandibular (or subangular) incision for exposure of the mandibular ramus
2. Condylar resection and coronoid resection (if indicated)
3. Shift of the mandible to the planned position, intermediate splint, intermaxillary fixation
4. Placement of total joint prosthesis and fixation by screws on both sides
5. Pack fat graft around articulation area of prosthesis (harvest fat from abdomen)
6. Close extraoral incisions
7. Remove intermaxillary fixation, intermediate splint
8. Maxillary osteotomies and mobilization
9. Intranasal procedures, if indicated (turbinectomies, nasal septoplasty, etc.)
10. Placement of final splint, intermaxillary fixation
11. Fixation of maxillary osteotomies by mini-plates (bone grafting, if indicated)
12. Removal of intermaxillary fixation, final splint
13. Close intraoral incisions

5.2 Unilateral TMJ reconstruction, split sagittal osteotomy on the contralateral side, with possible subsequent maxillary surgery

1. Endaural incision for exposure of the TMJ fossa and retromandibular (or subangular) incision for exposure of the mandibular ramus
2. Condylar resection and coronoid resection (if indicated)
3. Contralateral mandibular ramus sagittal split osteotomy
4. Shift of the mandible to the planned position, intermediate splint, intermaxillary fixation
5. Placement of total joint prosthesis and fixation by screws on both sides
6. Pack fat graft around articulation area of prosthesis (harvest fat from abdomen)
7. Close extraoral incisions
8. Rigid fixation to contralateral mandibular ramus osteotomy

9. Removal of intermaxillary fixation, intermediate splint

10. Maxillary osteotomies and mobilization

11. Intranasal procedures, if indicated (turbinectomies, nasal septoplasty, etc.)

12. Placement of final splint, intermaxillary fixation

13. Fixation of maxillary osteotomies by mini-plates (bone grafting, if indicated)

14. Removal of intermaxillary fixation, final splint

15. Close intraoral incisions

Note 1: For mandibular advancement or CCW rotation of the mandible, it is advisable to thoroughly relax the masticatory muscles. TJR surgery usually involves stripping the masseter muscle and detaching the lateral pterygoid muscle through condylectomy. In the case of coronoidectomy, the ligament of the temporal muscle is detached. In case of more extensive mandibular repositioning, the authors recommend detaching the pterygomasseteric sling at the edge of the mandible and stripping the lower part of the medial pterygoid muscle from the inner surface of the mandibular ramus (within 1 cm above the edge of the mandible).

Note 2: There is a different algorithm for performing orthognathic surgery with TJR in patients with ankylosis. Unless performing surgery only or surgery first, then patients with ankylosis will first undergo an ankylosis resection. This allows the mobilization of the jaw and at the same time allows the start of orthodontic preparation. Only after this is completed is orthognathic surgery performed, together with TJR. Spacers are inserted into the resected ankylosis site (most often bone cement) to prevent reankylosis.

6. Postoperative regimen and care, follow-up system

The postoperative regimen fundamentally differs depending on the scope of the surgery.

If mandibular repositioning is performed using bilateral TJR without maxillary surgery, then the postoperative regimen consists of [13, 16]:

1. Early rehabilitation of mouth opening – from the 1st day after surgery (when the pressure dressing is removed). For the first two weeks the patient opens his/her mouth freely to the point of pain, from the 3rd week the mouth is opened with the help of the fingers or a dilator to achieve a minimum opening of 35 mm- interincisively. Gentle massages of the masticatory muscles (several times a day) are recommended.

2. Antibiotics are administered for a period of 10 days (the first 3 days intravenously, then orally)

3. Analgesics are administered according to pain

4. Anti-edematous therapy is advised for the first 3 days

In patients where TJR is performed concurrently with SSO or maxillary surgery, the postoperative regimen consists of [13, 16]:

1. Intermaxillary fixation with elastic bands for a period of 6 weeks. The patient is instructed how to change the elastic bands and changes them twice daily – the patient uses this time to thoroughly clean the oral cavity and to freely open his/her mouth to the point of pain for at least 5 minutes. Gentle massage of the masticatory muscles (several times a day) are recommended.

2. Antibiotics are administered for a period of 10 days (the first 3 days intravenously, then orally)

3. Analgesics are administered according to pain

4. Anti-edematous therapy is advised for the first 3 days

Patients at the authors' workplace are typically hospitalized for several days after the surgery. In case of orthognathic surgery with TJR of the TMJ, hospitalization time is 3–7 days.

After surgery, each patient is scheduled for regular follow-up examinations at the authors' workplace at 2 weeks, one month, three months, 6 and 12 months after the procedure, and then regularly once a year after that [13].

Note 1: The authors prefer individual rehabilitation that largely relies on the patient's cooperation. The patient is instructed in methods for the rehabilitation of mouth opening and gentle muscle massages. If this rehabilitation is insufficient, a specialist, a physiotherapist, is brought in to help. The authors recommend specialized physiotherapy in case of complications – e.g., involvement of the facial nerve, trigeminal nerve [13].

Note 2: The risk of anterior dislocation of the prosthesis is increased due to the detachment of the ligaments of the masticatory muscles from the mandible (especially if a coronoidectomy was performed at the same time). It is appropriate to test the maximum range of motion of the mandible at the end of the surgery and to record whether or not dislocation occurs during maximal abduction [17]. If there is a risk of dislocation, temporary intermaxillary fixation with elastic bands is maintained (usually for the first postoperative week) [15].

7. Complications

We can divide complications into those associated with TJR and complications associated with orthognathic surgery.

Complications associated with TJR of the TMJ can be divided into perioperative and postoperative [15, 20, 34–37].

Perioperative complications include:

1. Injuries to blood vessels and nerves. Vessels mainly include the temporal superficial vein and artery, the retromandibular vein and branches of the maxillary artery. Of the nerves, the facial nerve can be damaged most often (manifested by impaired facial expressions in the postoperative period). Another damaged nerve may be the trigeminal nerve (manifested in the postoperative period by chronic pain, hypoesthesia or anesthesia of the lower lip area).

2. Injuries to surrounding anatomical regions - most often the external auditory canal, more rarely the structures of the middle ear

3. Poor insertion, inadequate fixation of prosthesis components

Postoperative complications include:

1. Surgical site infections – this can occur early (within 3 weeks of surgery, manifesting as swelling, redness of the surgical site, increased pain) or with a delay (more than 3 weeks after surgery, manifesting as diffuse swelling and pain, without erythema, fever). Wolford [36] reports early infectious complications due to oral flora, and late complications due to skin flora. The risk of infection increases with the amount and type of resident skin bacteria, nutritional factors, systemic disease, and habits.

2. Complicated healing of surgical wounds, unaesthetic scars

3. Dislocation of the condylar components of the prosthesis (**Figure 5**). The most common is anterior dislocation, which occurs due to weakening of masticatory muscle tension, especially when the temporal muscle is detached during coronoidectomy. We also encounter posterior condylar dislocations, especially in major mandibular advancements, due to the traction of suprahyoid muscles. A fossa prosthesis designed with a posterior shield can prevent posterior dislocation

4. Loosening of prosthesis components, failure of prosthesis material

5. Allergic reaction to prosthesis material

6. Heterotopic bone ossification - development of heterotopic bone around the prosthesis leading to limited jaw function, pain

7. Chronic pain. This occurs as a result of nerve injuries during surgery, infection of prosthesis components, loosening of the prosthesis, formation of heterotopic bone around the TJR or the fixation of chronic pain already present before the surgery.

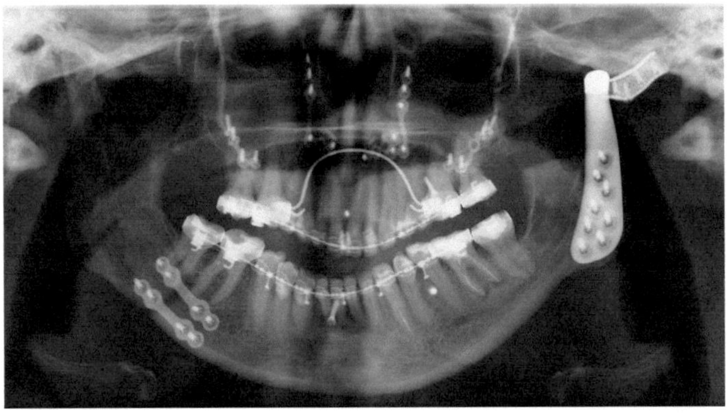

Figure 5.
Complication of TJR: luxation of prosthesis.

Complications associated with orthognathic surgery can again be divided into perioperative and postoperative [38, 39].

Perioperative complications include

1. Injuries to blood vessels-bleeding from the inferior alveolar artery, plexus pterygoideus, arteria palatina descendens, arteria maxillaris. The descending palatine artery is the most common source of mild to moderate bleeding during LeFort I osteotomy and subsequent delayed bleeding. Damage of the descending palatine artery may occur during medial wall osteotomy

2. Nerve injury - nervus alevolaris inferior, mental nerve, nervus palatinus major. Neurosensory alterations are normally perceived in the immediate postoperative period. They are the result of traction of the infraorbital nerve and direct trauma to the anterior, medial, and posterior superior alveolar nerves, as well as to the nasopalatine nerve and the descending palatal nerve

3. Bad split- unfavorable fracture

4. Inadequate mobilization of fragments

5. Tooth and periodontal damage in case of an inappropriate osteotomy line. An osteotomy closer than 5 mm to the dental apices poses the risk of root injuries.

6. Oronasal communication - mainly arises during the division of the maxilla into segments

Postoperative complications include

1. Bleeding (arteriovenous fistulae) can cause symptoms such as facial swelling, delayed bleeding, and development of a pulsatile sof mass

2. Neurosensory deficit- osteotomy induces changes in the maxillary teeth, buccal mucosa, palatal mucosa, and facial skin sensation. While skin sensation tends to recoer ovr time even after direct damage to sensory nerves, it may not completely recover to the condition that was present before surgery

3. Relapse

4. Delayed union or nonunion- of an osteotomy site may occur as a result of poor ealing of hard and soft tissues. The risk of nonunion is high when inadequate fixation is performed

5. Nasal septal malposition, which occurs after LeFort osteotomy and maxillary fixation. Septal malposition can occur during LeFort osteotomy and cause nasal deviation. The position of the septum must be checked, especially after extubation of the patient.

6. Inflammatory complications of the maxillary sinus

7. Release of osteosynthetic material

8. Infection Postoperative infections include cellulitis, abscess, maxillary sinusitis and osteomyelitis. Rates of postoperative infections are low thanks to aseptic techniques, antibiotics, and good blood supply into oral and maxillofacial area. Even when infections do occur, thex can be fully cured through early diagnosis and management.

8. Stability and assessment of the results of orthognathic surgery and TJR

If the quality or absence of joint structures does not ensure the stability of the result of orthognathic surgery, the combination with TJR guarantees a stable long-term result. The authors can confirm this from their own experience: 37 patients underwent orthognathic surgery concurrently with TJR (8 men, 29 women, average age 37, 1 years)- no relapse of DFD was recorded for at least one year after surgery (**Figures 6–19**).

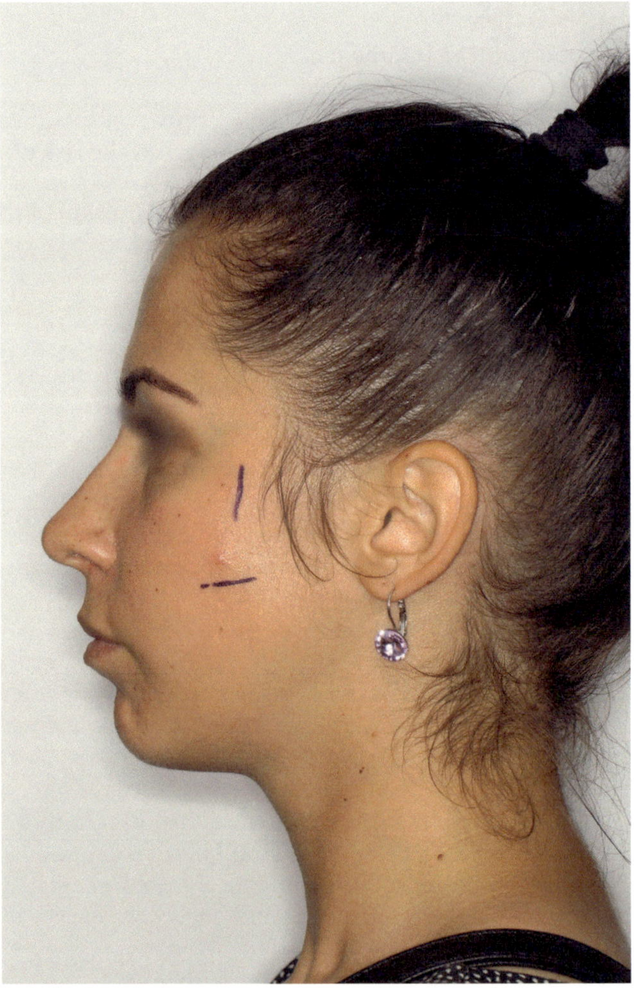

Figure 6.
28 years old woman with rheumatoid arthritis.

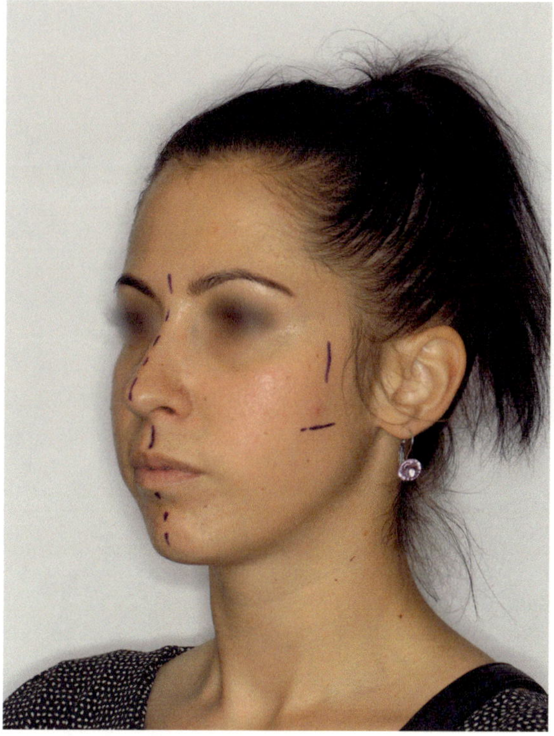

Figure 7.
28 years old woman with rheumatoid arthritis- before surgery.

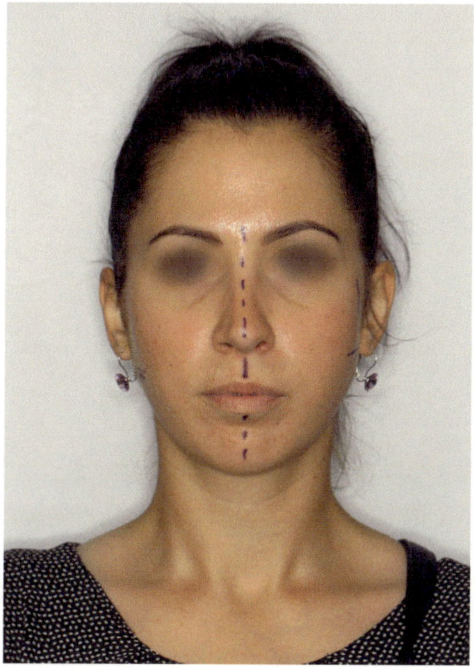

Figure 8.
28 years old woman with rheumatoid arthritis- frontal view.

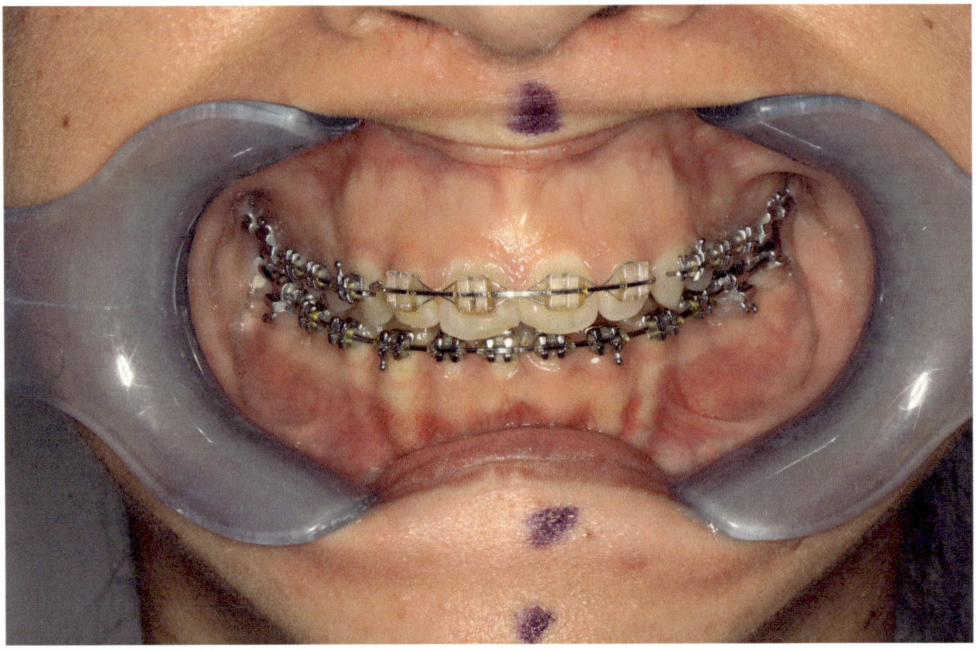

Figure 9.
28 years old woman with rheumatoid arthritis- occlusion before surgery.

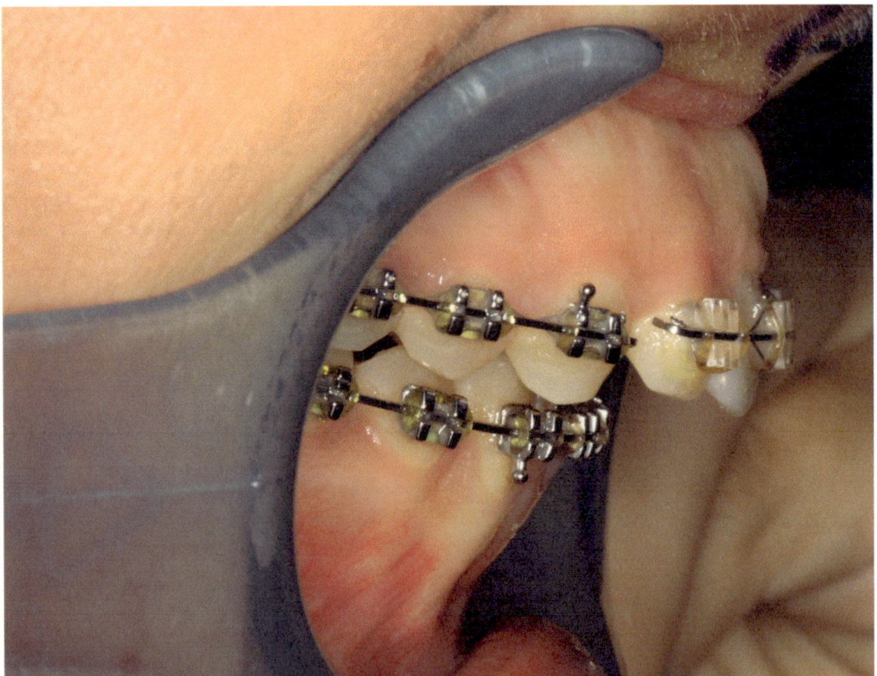

Figure 10.
28 years old woman with rheumatoid arthritis- occlusion before surgery, side view.

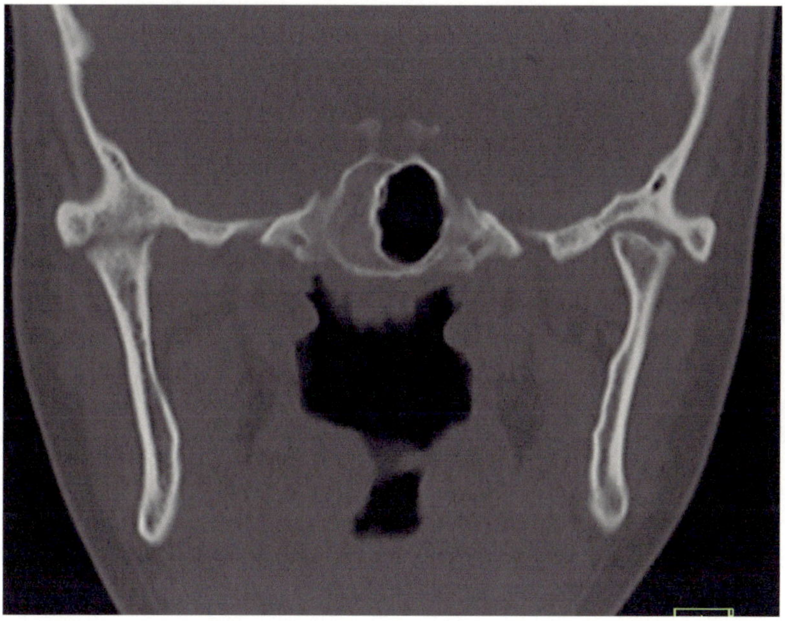

Figure 11.
CT scan with changes of TMJs.

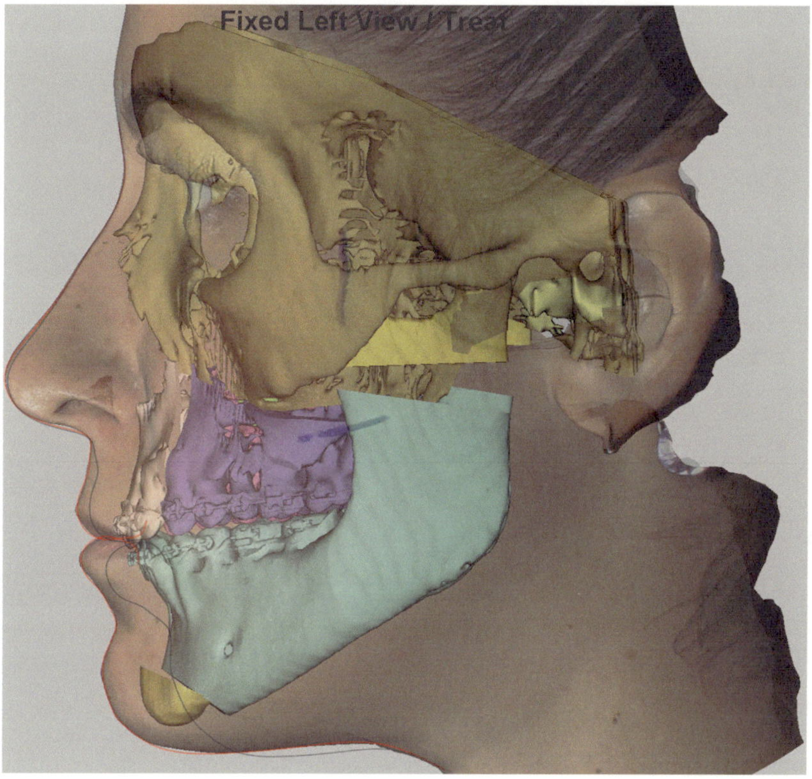

Figure 12.
28 years old woman with rheumatoid arthritis- Virtual planning.

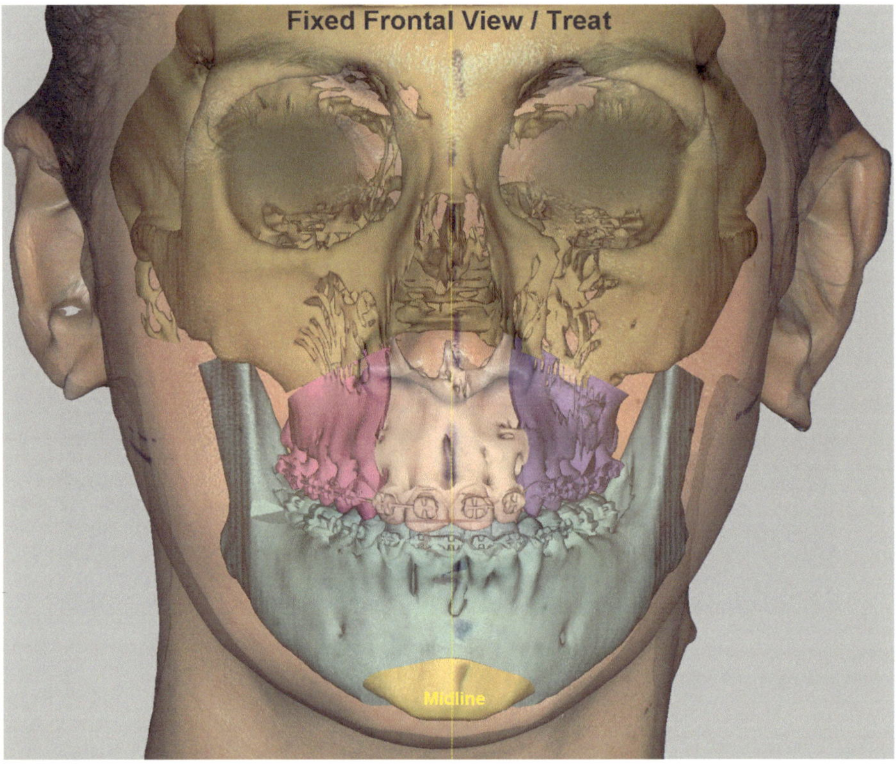

Figure 13.
28 years old woman with rheumatoid arthritis- Virtual planning, frontal view.

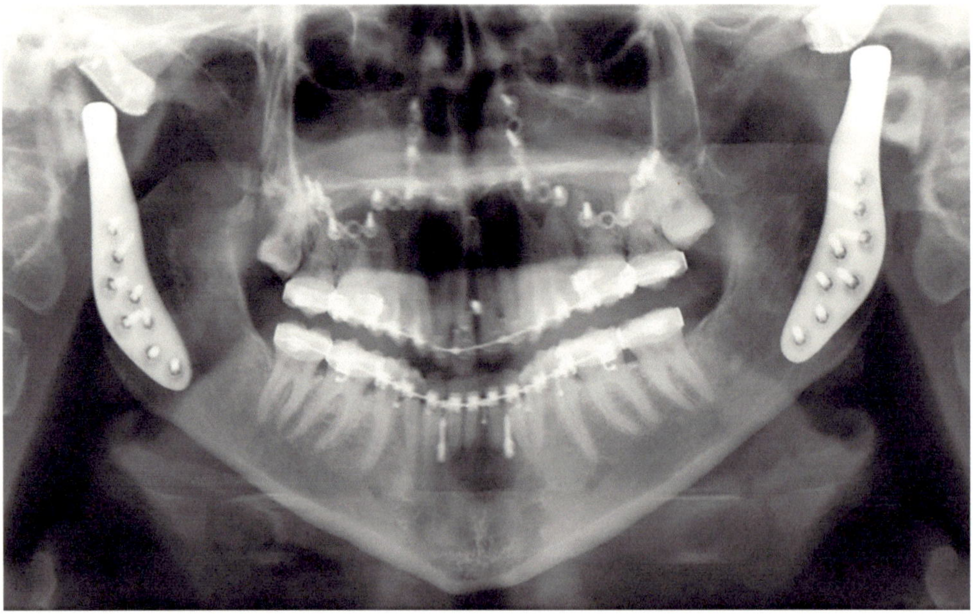

Figure 14.
28 years old woman with rheumatoid arthritis- X ray after orthognatic surgery and TJR of TMJs.

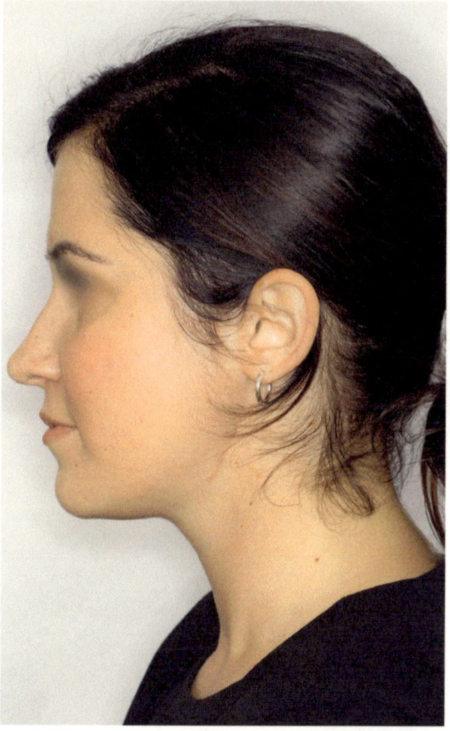

Figure 15.
28 years old woman with rheumatoid arthritis- after surgery- side view.

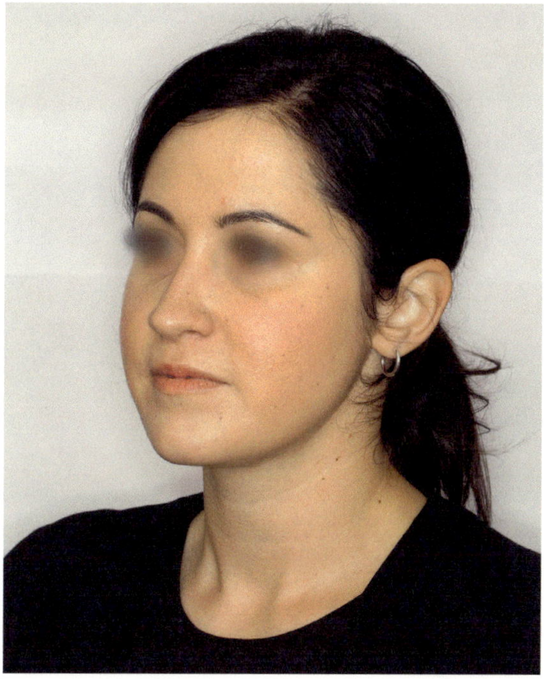

Figure 16.
28 years old woman with rheumatoid arthritis- after surgery.

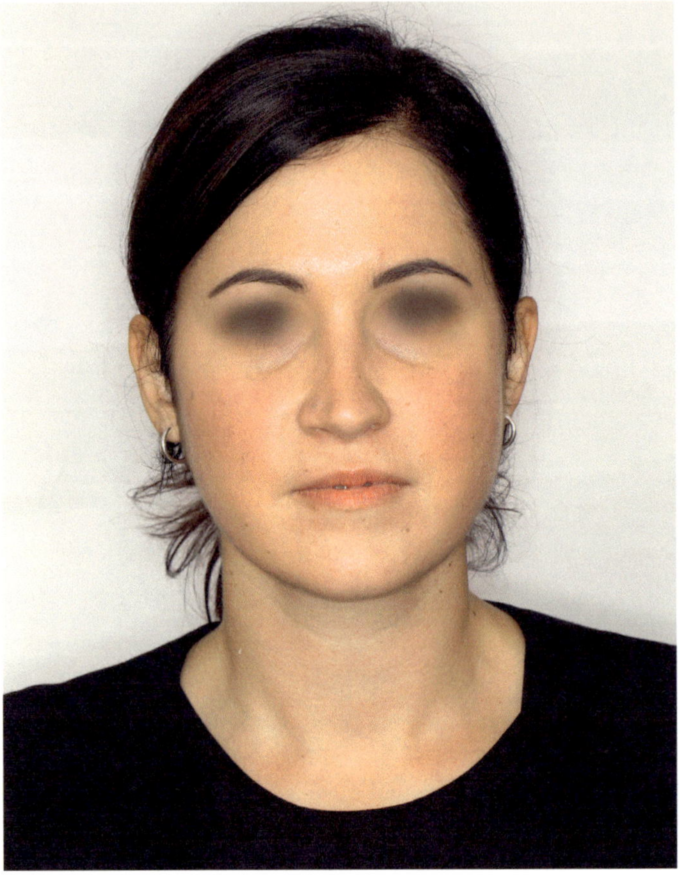

Figure 17.
28 years old woman with rheumatoid arthritis- after surgery- frontal view.

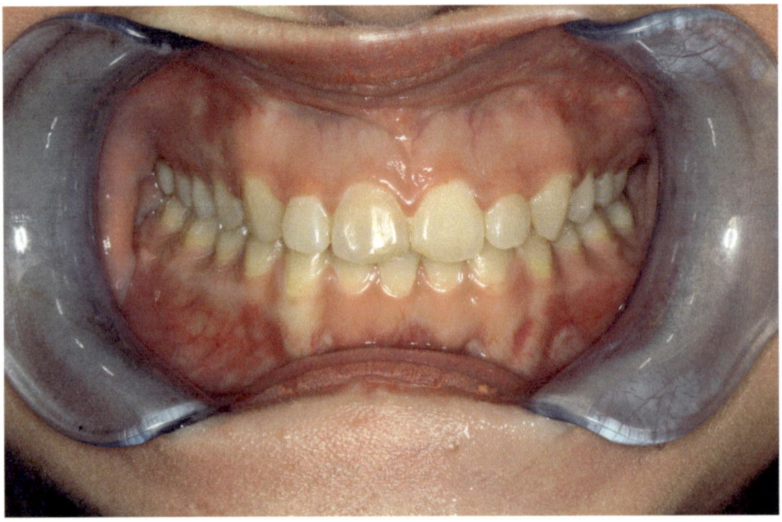

Figure 18.
28 years old woman with rheumatoid arthritis- occlusion after surgery.

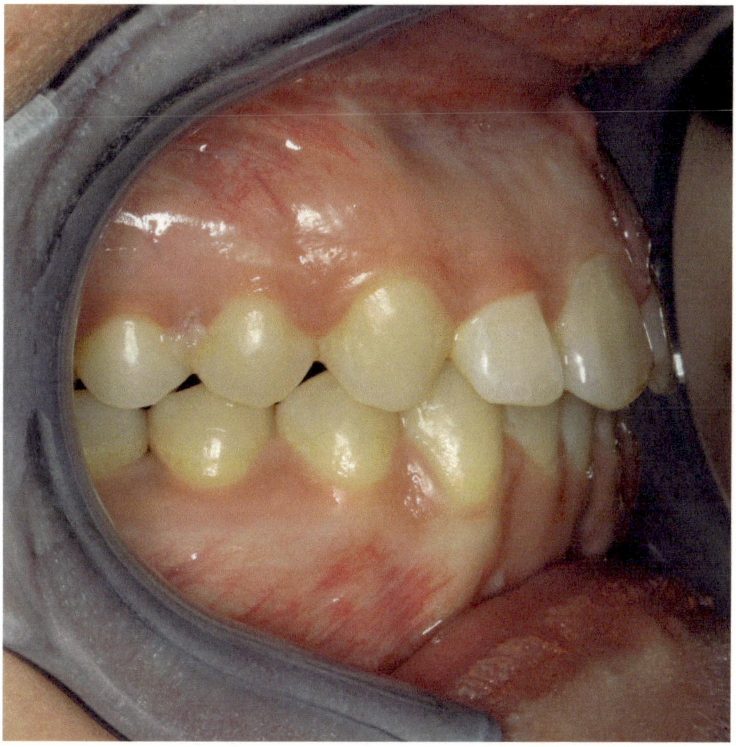

Figure 19.
28 years old woman with rheumatoid arthritis- occlusion after surgery, side view.

A number of authors have confirmed this fact in their studies [2, 11, 40–42] both in the stability of CCW rotation associated with TJR [40] and in the number of TMJ pathologies: autoimmune diseases with TMJ - rheumatoid arthritis and juvenile idiopathic arthritis [41], HFM [11], ICR [42].

9. Conclusion, summary

A stable TMJ without signs of pathology is a basic prerequisite for successful orthognathic surgery. If pathology is present, it is necessary to first address the condition of the TMJ (through conservative, mini-invasive and surgical methods). Only after the condition of the TMJ is stabilized is it possible to surgically address DFD.

In the indicated conditions (reduced joint function due to pathological changes of the condyle, reduction of condyle height due to pathological processes in the TMJ, absence of the condyle, TMJ ankylosis or previous unsatisfactory surgical therapy), it is necessary to replace joint structures. Allogeneic patient-fitted prostheses are ideally used for TMJ reconstruction, as the shape of these prostheses allows the lower jaw to be moved to the appropriate position.

Orthognathic surgery in conjunction with TJR is performed in a single operation, where precise planning of these surgical procedures is vital for their successful execution. The patient's cooperation during postoperative care is also an integral part of successful orthognathic surgery with TJR.

Personal thanks

Authors thank to Medika Trade Praha for support.

Author details

Vladimír Machoň* and Michal Beňo
Department of Oral Maxillofacial Surgery, Charles University and Faculty Hospital Prague, Czech Republic

*Address all correspondence to: machonv@seznam.cz

References

[1] Wolford LM, Concomitant TMJ. Total joint replacement and orthognatic surgery. Chapter 6. In: Meruri LG, editor. Temporomandibular joint replacement. Switzerland: Springer International Publisher; 2016. pp. 133-163

[2] Matthews S, Hechler BL, Shah R. Reprint of The Role of Total Joint Replacement Surgery in the Orthognathic Patient. Seminars in Orthodontics. 2021;**27**(10):286-293

[3] Mercuri LG, Wolford LM, Sanders B, White RD, Hurder A, Henderson W. Custom CAD/CAM total temporomandibular joint reconstruction system: Preliminary multicenter report. Journal of Oral and Maxillofacial Surgery. 1995;**53**:106-115

[4] Wolford LM. Computer-assisted surgical simulation for concomitant temporomandibular joint custom-fitted total joint reconstruction and orthognathic surgery. Atlas of the Oral and Maxillofacial Surgery Clinics of North America. 2016;**24**:55-66

[5] Sembronio S, Tel A, Robiony M. Protocol for fully digital and customized management of concomitant temporomandibular joint replacement and orthognathic surgery. International Journal of Oral and Maxillofacial Surgery. 2021;**50**:212-219

[6] Movahed R, Teschke M, Wolford LM. Protocol for concomitant temporomandibular joint custom-fitted total joint reconstruction and orthognathic surgery utilizing computer-assisted surgical simulation. Journal of Oral and Maxillofacial Surgery. 2013;**71**:2123-2129

[7] Gupta RJ, Silva R, Connelly ST. Bilateral temporomandibular joint reconstruction and maxillomandibular advancement for concomitant temporomandibular joint degeneration and obstructive sleep apnea. Atlas of the Oral and Maxillofacial Surgery Clinics of North America. 2019;**27**:43-52

[8] Gunson MJ, Arnett GW, Milam SB. Pathophysiology and pharmacologic control of osseous mandibular condylar resorption. Journal of Oral and Maxillofacial Surgery. 2012;**70**(8): 1918-1934

[9] Wolford LM, Cardenas L. Idiopathic condylar resorption: Diagnosis, treatment protocol, and outcomes. American Journal of Orthodontics and Dentofacial Orthopedics. 1999;**116**(6):667-677

[10] Mercuri LG, Handelman CS. Idiopathic Condylar Resorption: What Should We Do? Oral and Maxillofacial Surgery Clinics of North America. 2020;**32**(1):105-116

[11] Wolford LM, Campbell Bourland T, Rodrigues D, Perez DE, Limoeiro E. Successful reconstruction of nongrowing hemifacial microsomia patients with unilateral temporomandibular joint total joint prosthesis and orthognathic surgery. Journal of Oral and Maxillofacial Surgery. 2012;**70**:2835-2853

[12] Kummoona R. Biological reconstruction of the temporomandibular joint by chondro-osseous graft: clinical and experimental study. The Journal of Craniofacial Surgery. 2013 May;**24**(3):792-796

[13] Machoň V. Manual of TMJ Surgery. The Prague approaches. Prague: Business Media Publishing; 2017. p. 111

[14] Mercuri LG. The use of alloplastic prostheses for temporomandibular joint

reconstruction. Journal of Oral and Maxillofacial Surgery. 2000;**58**:70-75

[15] Meruri LG, editor. Temporomandibular joint replacement. A comprehensive reference for researschers, materials, scientists and surgeons. Switzerland: Springer International Publisher; 2016. p. 301

[16] Giannakopoulos HE, Sinn DP, Quinn PD. Biomet Microfixation Temporomandibular Joint Replacement System: A 3-year follow-up study of patients treated during 1995 to 2005. Journal of Oral and Maxillofacial Surgery. 2012;**70**(4):787-794

[17] Sidebottom AJ, Gruber E. One-year prospective outcome analysis and complications following total replacement of the temporomandibular joint with the TMJ Concepts system. The British Journal of Oral & Maxillofacial Surgery. 2013;**51**:620-624

[18] Gomez NL, Boccalatte LA, Lopez Ruiz Á, Nassif MG, Figari MF, Ritacco L. Total temporomandibular joint replacement and simultaneous orthognathic surgery using computer-assisted surgery. J Maxillofac Oral Surg. 2021;**20**(3):394-403

[19] Quinn PD. Lorenz prosthesis. In: Donlon WC, editor. Total temporomandibular joint reconstruction, Oral and Maxillofacial Surgery Clinics of North America. Vol. 12. Philadelphia: W. B. Saunders; 2000. pp. 93-104

[20] Yadav P, Roychoudhury A, Kumar RD, Bhutia O, Bhutia T, Aggarwal B. Total Alloplastic Temporomandibular Joint Replacement. J Maxillofac Oral Surg. 2021;**20**(4):515-526

[21] Mercuri LG, Swift JQ. Considerations for the use of alloplastic temporomandibular joint replacement in the growing patient. Journal of Oral and Maxillofacial Surgery. 2009;**67**:1979-1990

[22] Sinn DP, Tandon R, Tiwana PS. Can alloplastic total temporomandibular joint reconstruction be used in the growing patient? A preliminary report. Journal of Oral and Maxillofacial Surgery. 2021;**79**(11):2267-2267

[23] Collins CP, Wilson KJ, Collins PC. Lateral pterygoid myotomy with reattachment to the condylar neck: An adjunct to restore function after total joint reconstruction. Oral Surgery, Oral Medicine, Oral Pathology, Oral Radiology, and Endodontics. 2003;**95**:672-679

[24] Mommaerts MY. On the reinsertion of the lateral pterygoid tendon in total temporomandibular joint replacement surgery. Journal of Cranio-Maxillo-Facial Surgery. 2019;**47**:1913-1917

[25] Tamburrino RK, Boucher NS, Vanarsdall RL, Secchi AG. The transverse dimension: Diagnosis and relevance to functional occlusion. RWISO J. 2010;**2**(1):13-21

[26] Cintra O, Grybauskas S, Vogel CJ, Latkauskiene D, Gama NA Jr. Digital platform for planning facial asymmetry orthodontic-surgical treatment preparation. Dental Press J Orthod. 2018;**23**(3):80-93

[27] Liou EJW, Chen PS, Wang YC, Yu CC, Huang CS, Chen YR. Surgery-first accelerated orthognathic surgery: postoperative rapid orthodontic tooth movement. Journal of Oral and Maxillofacial Surgery. 2011;**69**:781-785

[28] Liao YF, Chiu YT, Huang CS, Ko EW, Chen YR. Presurgical orthodontics versus no presurgical orthodontics: treatment outcome of surgicalorthodontic correction for skeletal class III open bite. Plastic and Reconstructive Surgery. 2010;**126**:2074-2083

[29] McCormick SU, Drew SJ. Virtual model surgery for efficient planning and surgical performance. Journal of Oral and Maxillofacial Surgery. 2011;**69**(3):638-644

[30] Herna'ndez-Alfaro F, Guijarro-Martı'nez R. On a definition of the appropriate timing for surgical intervention in orthognathic surgery. International Journal of Oral and Maxillofacial Surgery. 2014;**43**(7):846-855

[31] Pelo S, Gasparini G, Garagiola U, Cordaro M, Di Nardo F, Staderini. Surgery-first orthognathic approach vs traditional orthognathic approach: oral health-related quality of life assessed with 2 questionnaires. American Journal of Orthodontics and Dentofacial Orthopedics. 2017;**152**:250-254

[32] Perez DE, Garza R Jr. Computer-assisted design and manufacturing in combined orthognathic and temporomandibular joint surgery. Atla Oral Maxillofacial Surg Clin North Am. 2020;**28**(2):83-93

[33] Haas OL Jr, Becker OE, Oliveira RB. Computer-aided planning in orthognathic surgery—systematic review. International Journal of Oral and Maxillofacial Surgery. 2015;**44**:329-342

[34] Gruber EA, McCullough J, Sidebottom AJ. Medium-term outcomes and complications after total replacement of the temporomandibular joint. Prospective outcome analysis after 3 and 5 years. The British Journal of Oral & Maxillofacial Surgery. 2015;**53**(5):412-415

[35] Murdoch B, Buchanan J, Cliff J. Temporomandibular joint replacement: A New Zealand perspective. International Journal of Oral and Maxillofacial Surgery. 2014;**43**(5):595-599

[36] Wolford LM, Rodrigues DB, McPhillips A. Management of the infected temporomandibular joint total joint prosthesis. Journal of Oral and Maxillofacial Surgery. 2010;**68**:2810-2823

[37] Machon V, Levorova J, Hirjak D, Drahos M, Brizman E, Beno M, et al. Evaluation of complications following stock replacement of the temporomandibular joint performed between the years 2006 and 2015: A retrospective study. Oral and Maxillofacial Surgery. 2020;**24**(3):373-379

[38] Tabrizi R., Mohammad HM. Complications of Orthognatic Surgery. In: A textbook of Advanced Oral and Maxillofacial Surgery, volume 3, London United Kingdom: Intech Open, 2016 (online)

[39] Kim YK. Complications associated with orthognatic surgery. Journal of the Korean Association of Oral and Maxillofacial Surgeons. 2017;**43**(1):3-15

[40] Dela Coleta KE, Wolford LM, Gonçalves JR, Pinto Ados S, Pinto LP, Cassano DS. Maxillo-mandibular counter-clockwise rotation and mandibular advancement with TMJ Concepts total joint prostheses: part I--skeletal and dental stability. International Journal of Oral and Maxillofacial Surgery. 2009;**38**(2):126-138

[41] Wolford LM, Kesterke MJ. Does Combined Temporomandibular Joint Reconstruction With Patient-Fitted Total Joint Prosthesis and Orthognathic Surgery Provide Stable Skeletal and Occlusal Outcomes in Juvenile Idiopathic Arthritis Patients? Journal of Oral and Maxillofacial Surgery. 2022;**80**(1):138-150

[42] Mehra P, Nadershah M, Chigurupati R. Is alloplastic temporomandibular joint reconstruction a viable option in the surgical management of adult patients with idiopathic condylar resorption? Journal of Oral and Maxillofacial Surgery. 2016;**74**:2044-2054

Chapter 4

Alloplastic TMJ Reconstruction

Sundaram Ravanasamudram Rajaram, Gauthami Sundar and Rajaram Ravanasamudram Sundaram

Abstract

Total Alloplastic Temporomandibular joint reconstruction has been the treatment of choice for extreme cases of Temporomandibular Joint Disease and Pathology. Some of the remarkable advantages that are enjoyed with this device are early functional restoration, long term stability and improved jaw function. The prosthesis can be custom made to the particular individual also. This chapter provides an insight of the basics of Total Alloplastic Temporomandibular joint reconstruction which is evidence based.

Keywords: temporomandibular joint, alloplastic TMJ reconstruction, TMJ anatomy, comparative anatomy TMJ, 3D reconstruction

1. Introduction

The need for the joint prosthesis comes up with the severity of the joint pathology. Failure of conservative therapies and non-surgical management, and surgical procedures with limited success rates leading to recurrence of the disease form the background for the development of the total alloplastic device for Temporomandibular Joint (TMJ).

The main goal of the reconstruction is to restore the form and function [1] of the jaw. In the yesteryears, Autogenous bones were used in most cases of Temporpmandibular Joint Reconstruction (TMJR). Revision surgeries in cases of TMJR with costochondral grafts need to be considered keeping in mind its excessive growth potential. The autogenous bone in growing individuals pose significant risks that may impair the jaw anatomy and function on a long run frequently leading to readdressing the joint problem. Innumerable evidence now exists in favour of the total joint replacement procedure where the joint anatomy and function being restored focussing more on the Biomechanical aspects [2].

Emerging studies support TMJR in terms of improved quality of life, improved masticatory function, improved jaw movement, speech and anatomy [3–5].

The device is made up of Cobalt-Chrome-Molybdenum (Co-Cr-Mo) or Titanium (Ti) condylar components with ultrahigh molecular weight polyethylene (UHMWPE) owing to their inert and bio friendly nature. These implants are available as stock fit and custom made that are patient specific.

On reviewing the literature, in the field of alloplastic TMJR, is interesting in that in 1974, Kiehn et al. attempted to construct an alloplastic TMJR prosthesis which was based on the principle used for total hip replacement with vitallium fossa and condyle unit.

In 1982, the vitek- Kent proplast—Teflon (PT) containing process was created (Vitek, Inc., Houston, Texas). What was initially successful was found to be a failure in a long run. In 1989 custom fit total TMJR system based on CAD CAM data was introduced by Techmedia that continues to be successful as of now [6].

In any TMJR, to be successful, some of the biological and mechanical characteristics are to be considered [7–9].

1. It should simulate the movements of TMJ

2. It should have close adaptability

3. Vivo longevity with regards to simulation of TMJ movements offering perfect imitation of translational movement of condyle without restricting the movements of uninvolved non replaced contralateral joint

4. Choosing a material with appropriate mechanical properties, tensile strength, hardness, elasticity and fatigue coefficience that will prevent stress from being transferred to adjacent bones, which may cause bone resorption and implant loosening.

1.1 Comparative anatomy pertaining to TMJ

The TMJ of mammals is different from other vertebrates, interestingly for functional modifications in that the articulating disc arose as a tendon which became pinched by the joint that is originated by intramembranous bones. Hence the growth depends on cartilaginous structures [10–12].

The TMJ anatomy size, shape, type of movements, and the load that it can take are species specific such as loss of synovial cavities in whales, loss of primary absence of disc in marsupials (sloths), variation in orientation of joint cavity in rodents, reversal of usual convex concave relationship to turn the mandibular condyle into a female element in sheeps and cattle, size variation and higher loading or lower loading depending on its pre requirement. Eg: crocodiles [13].

Sliding or side to side movement is also a variant. Considering all the animals, the human being's TMJ anatomy has the most evolved anatomical structures for efficient masticatory function for present day.

1.2 Anatomy of TMJ

The TMJ is a synovial joint of condylar variety [14]. It is also known as ginglimo arthrodial joint. It has two compartments namely the upper joint space and lower joint space lined by cartilaginous cells and divided by a fibrocartilaginous disc.

The upper bony component is formed by the temporal bone and the lower articulating joint is formed by the head of the condylar process of the mandible. The joint cavity is encapsulated by a fibrous capsule that is filled with the synovial fluid. The disc is held in position by the discal ligaments and the lateral pterygoid insertion.

This attachment leads to certain disorders like clicking joint and so on and so surgical anatomy of TMJ should be studied at length before analysing the pathology.

The ligaments supporting the TMJ can be classified into intracapsular and extracapsular.

The intracapsular ligaments are the capsule, the interdiscal ligaments.

The extracapsular ligaments are the ligament of TMJ, stylomandibular ligament and sphenomandibular ligament.

1.3 Freakishness of TMJ

Anatomical considerations of freakishness of TMJ [15] pertaining to healing of alloplastic reconstruction are interesting in that these qualities are not met with in other joints of humankind.

Non weight bearing aspect of TMJ is peculiar. The function of TMJ on one side depends considerably on the health of other side TMJ and occlusal apparatus. This tripartiate relationship is very useful at times and also troublesome while treating TMJ pathologies with alloplastic TMJR.

Abundant vascular supply for the TMJ is any another unique feature. What triggers excellent tendency to heal in comparison with other joint procedures is yet not clearly understood so the whole focus in alloplastic grafting is to limit excessive post-surgical ankyloses to make it success.

1.4 Indications for TMJ alloplastic joints

The decision to take up TMJR [16, 17] has been suggested by various organisations such as national institute of health and care excellence (NICE) in May 2014(8) and the British association of oral and maxillofacial surgeons in 2008(9). A few situations where alloplastic joint reconstruction is preferred are

1. Failed previous alloplastic and/ or autogenous joint reconstruction
2. post traumatic condylar injury
3. Avascular necrosis
4. Reconstruction after tumour ablative surgery
5. Developmental abnormalities
6. Functional deformities
7. Severe inflammatory condition that fail to respond to conservative treatment.
8. It is likely that the use of alloplastic TMJR will be on the increase in paediatric field since such surgery may significantly improve the quality of life and reduce many of the functional limitations.

1.5 Contraindications

Absolute contraindications for alloplastic TMJR are many in which primary consideration is active infection [18–21]. In acute infection if prosthesis is placed it can lead to micromotion and difficulty to stabilise the process and ultimately leading to failure. Next important contraindication is in those with documented allergy to implant components which may be present before or may manifest after the placement of prosthesis and are generally type IV delayed hypersensitivities.

Placement of fat grafts around the head of condylar components to decrease the tissue exposure to alloy components has been previously proposed by some authors and although this approach is reasonable there is no objective scientific evidence to support this hypothesis. Titanium prosthesis eliminate the possible allergy caused by Chromium cobalt Nickel Molebednum.

Uncontrolled systemic disease is considered yet another contraindication. A proper psychological preparation of preoperative evaluation must be considered essential particularly in elderly patients.

In a growing individual, alloplastic TMJR device necessitates reoperation.

1.6 Case report

A 20 years old male presented with Bilateral recurrent TMJ ankyloses (**Figure 1**). Initial TMJ injury was manged conservatively (2 years before) and hence no secondary deformities present. After some days he developed progressive Bilateral TMJ ankyloses. On clinical examination the mouth opening was 2 mm. Radiographic features showed development of radiopaque masses of Bilateral TMJ spaces with shortening of ramal height, signifying TMJ ankyloses. Bilateral TMJR with alloplastic device was planned.

1.7 Fabrication of the TMJ implant

Over a period of time, TMJ implants were facing menace due to excessive healing or ankyloses and hence fascia interposed osteoarthroplasty, muscle interposed osseoarthroplasty were carried out but were unsuccessfully (**Figure 2**).

Gap arthroplasty was reasonably successful but the anatomical disfigurement was experienced and hence metal implants were successfully (CO, Ti, Mb) used if allergic reactions were not a problem. At later stages titanium came into rescue to eliminate allergic reactions.

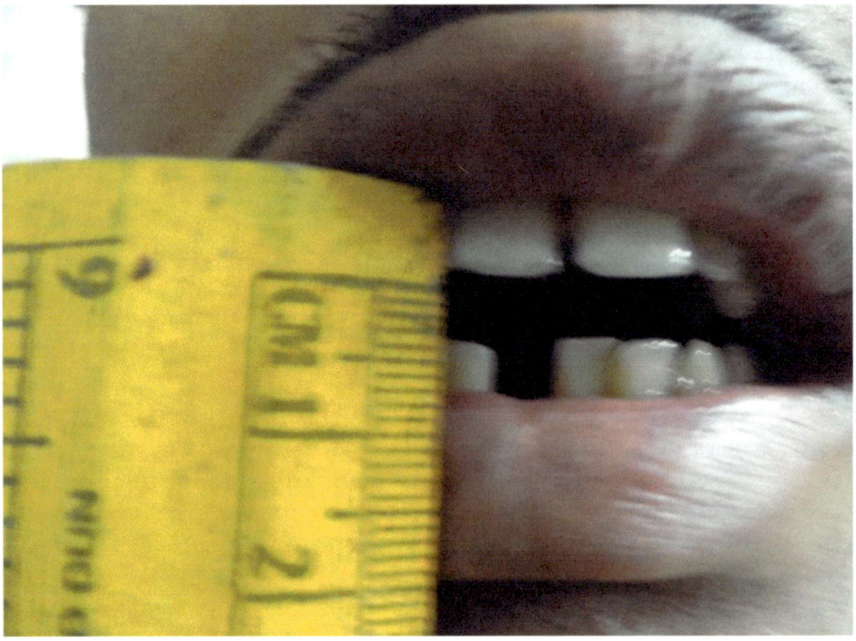

Figure 1.
Preoperative limited mouth opening.

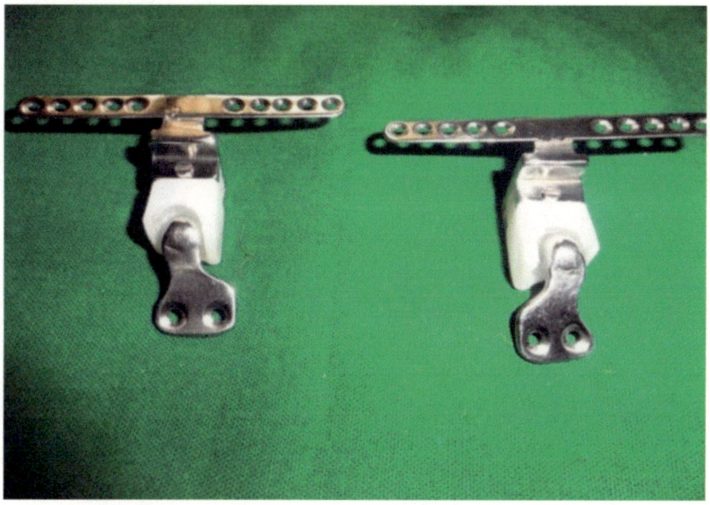

Figure 2.
Custom made TMJ alloplastic device.

Using such devices had some teething troubles.

1. The implants can be heavy causing discomfort to the patients. The Young's modulus of titanium is almost 5 times that of cortical bone and results in stress shielding effects [22, 23].

2. It is not cost effective and time consuming

The general difficulty all the surgeons experience were that the readymade implants did not have the ideal requisites of an implant as they do not snuggly fit.

Hence with the development of 3 D reconstruction digitally, the TMJR has come to near perfection.

The process involves making a CT for the patient and subsequent construction of Rapid prototyping (RP).

The resultant model involves the pathology of the TMJ (if any) which requires a trimming of the pathology in the model and 3D reconstruction of the implant digitally.

In this case, the prosthesis was patient specific. It consisted of the fossa and condylar components with the height of the device fabricated so as to compensate for the vertical height lost due to ramal shortening and gap arthroplasty.

The fossa eminence component articular surface was made of ultra-high-molecular-weight polyethylene over the stainless steel frame with 2 mm screw holes.

The stainless steel condylar unit has anteroposterior dimension of 5 mm and mediolateral dimension of 8 mm, with screw holes for fixation (**Figure 2**).

Intraoperative pictures show the snug fit of the prosthesis (**Figure 3a** and **b**).

Thus the main goal of the procedure was achieved viz., mouth opening and jaw function (**Figure 4**).

Postoperative check x ray was done to check for the proper positioning of the device (**Figure 5**).

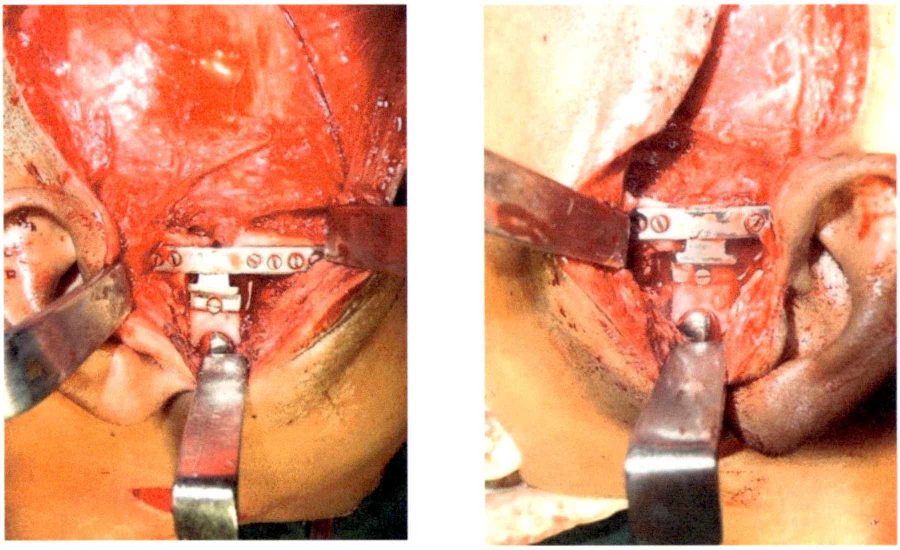

(a) (b)

Figure 3.
(a) TMJ alloplastic device in situ—Right side; and (b) TMJ alloplastic device in situ—Left side.

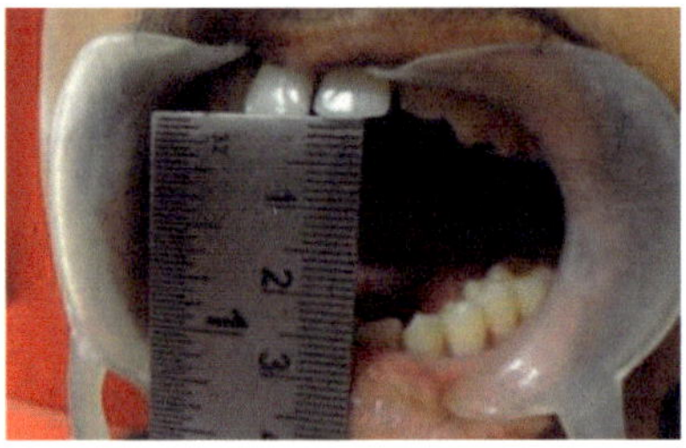

Figure 4.
Postoperative mouth opening.

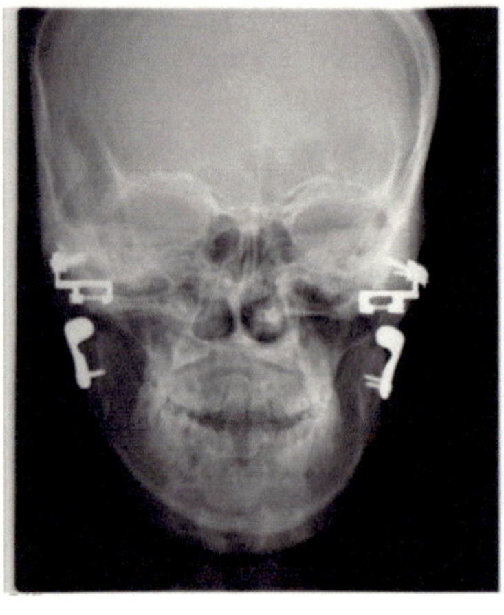

Figure 5.
Postoperative radiograph confirming the TMJ alloplastic device in situ.

2. Conclusion

Considering the possible disadvantages of autogenous reconstruction of TMJ like unpredictable growth potential and graft fracture the Alloplastic implants constitute a superior option by way of producing predictable healing and functional duplication. The previously mentioned defects of heaviness of the metal and cost effectiveness are the future challenges in the field of TMJR.

Acknowledgements

Dr. Neelakandan RS, Vice chancellor, MAHER University, Chennai, Tamil Nadu.

Conflict of interest

"The authors declare no conflict of interest."

Notes/thanks/other declarations

I extend my sincere thanks and gratitude to Dr. Gauthami Sundar and Dr. Rajaram for the timely support.

Author details

Sundaram Ravanasamudram Rajaram[1*], Gauthami Sundar[2] and Rajaram Ravanasamudram Sundaram[2]

1 International Medical Center, Fujairah, United Arab Emirates

2 Rajaram's Dental Surgery, India

*Address all correspondence to: sundarum88@gmail.com

References

[1] Mercuri LG. Alloplastic temporomandibular joint replacement: Rationale for the use of custom devices. International Journal of Oral and Maxillofacial Surgery. 2012;**41**(9):1033-1040

[2] Amstutz HC, Campbell P, Kossovsky N, Clarke IC. Mechanism and clinical significance of wear debris-induced osteolysis. Clinical Orthopaedics and Related Research. 1992;**276**:7-18

[3] Kunjur J, Niziol R, Matthews NS. Quality of life: Patient-reported outcomes after total replacement of the temporomandibular joint. The British Journal of Oral & Maxillofacial Surgery. 2016;**54**(7):762-766

[4] Mercuri LG, Edibam NR, Giobbie-Hurder A. Fourteen-year follow-up of a patient-fitted total temporomandibular joint reconstruction system. Journal of Oral and Maxillofacial Surgery. 2007;**65**(6):1140-1148

[5] Wolford LM, Mercuri LG, Schneiderman ED, Movahed R, Allen W. Twenty-year follow-up study on a patient-fitted temporomandibular joint prosthesis: The Techmedica/TMJ concepts device. Journal of Oral and Maxillofacial Surgery. 2015;**73**(5):952960

[6] Kiehn CL, DesPrez JD, Converse CF. A new procedure for total temporomandibular joint replacement. Plastic and Reconstructive Surgery. 1974;**53**(2):221-226

[7] Wolford LM, Mehra P. Custom-made total joint prostheses for temporomandibular joint reconstruction. Baylor University Medical Center Proceedings. 2000;**13**(2):135-138

[8] van Loon JP, de Bont GM, Boering G. Evaluation of temporomandibular joint prostheses: Review of the literature from 1946 to 1994 and implications for future prosthesis designs. Journal of Oral and Maxillofacial Surgery. 1995;**53**(9): 984-996; discussion 96-97

[9] van Loon JP, de Bont LG, Stegenga B, Spijkervet FK, Verkerke GJ. Groningen temporomandibular joint prosthesis. Development and first clinical application. International Journal of Oral and Maxillofacial Surgery. 2002;**31**(1):44-52

[10] Smith KK. The evolution of mammalian development. Bulletin of the Museum of Comparative Zoology at Harvard College. 2001;**156**:119-135

[11] Sprinz R. A note on the mandibular intra-articular disc in the joints of Marsupialia and Monotremata. Proceedings of the Zoological Society of London. 1965;**144**:327-338

[12] Du Brul EL. Evolution of the temporomandibular joint. In: Sarnat BG, editor. The Temporomandibular Joint. Springfield, IL: Charles C Thomas; 1964. pp. 3-27

[13] Scapino RP. The third joint of the canine jaw. Journal of Morphology. 1965;**116**:23-50

[14] Bordoni B, Varacallo M. Anatomy, Head and neck, temporomandibular joint. . In: StatPearls. Treasure Island (FL): StatPearls Publishing; 2022. Available from: https://www.ncbi.nlm.nih.gov/books/NBK538486/

[15] Herring SW. TMJ anatomy and animal models. Journal of Musculoskeletal & Neuronal Interactions. 2003;**3**(4):391

[16] Excellence. NIfHaC. Total Prosthetic Replacement of the Temporomandibular Joint: NICE Interventional Procedure Guidance 500. London: NICE; 2014

[17] Sidebottom AJ. surgeons UTr, British Association of O, maxillofacial S. guidelines for the replacement of temporomandibular joints in the United Kingdom. The British Journal of Oral & Maxillofacial Surgery. 2008;**46**(2):146-147

[18] Wolford LM, Dingwerth DJ, Talwar RM, Pitta MC. Comparison of 2 temporomandibular joint total joint prosthesis systems. Journal of Oral and Maxillofacial Surgery. 2003;**61**(6):685-690 discussion 90

[19] Wolford LM, Karras SC. Autologous fat transplantation around temporomandibular joint total joint prostheses: Preliminary treatment outcomes. Journal of Oral and Maxillofacial Surgery. 1997;**55**(3):245-251; discussion 51-52

[20] Hussain OT, Sah S, Sidebottom AJ. Prospective comparison study of one-year outcomes for all titanium total temporomandibular joint replacements in patients allergic to metal and cobalt-chromium replacement joints in patients not allergic to metal. The British Journal of Oral & Maxillofacial Surgery. 2014;**52**(1):34-37

[21] Mercuri LG, Swift JQ. Considerations for the use of alloplastic temporomandibular joint replacement in the growing patient. Journal of Oral and Maxillofacial Surgery. 2009;**67**(9):1979-1990

[22] Robertson DM, Pierre L, Chahal R. Preliminary observations of bone ingrowth into porous materials. Journal of Biomedical Materials Research. 1976;**10**:335-344

[23] Ryan G, Pandit A, Apatsidis D. Fabrication methods of porous metals for use in orthopedic applications. Biomaterials. 2006;**27**:2651-2670

Section 3

Various Techniques for Managements of TMJ Disease

Chapter 5

Biomechanics of the Temporomandibular Joint

Pablo Andrés Crespo Reinoso, Emilio Ruiz Delgado and James Jerez Robalino

Abstract

Biomechanics is the study of mechanics applied to living beings, it analyzes loads, stress, tension, movement, size, shape, and structure of the body. The temporomandibular joint in physiological states is subject to the interaction of various bone (jaw and temporal), nervous, cartilaginous, and muscular components. When there is an alteration in any of the components, normal biomechanics are affected. Knowing in detail how each element works individually and is essential for the diagnosis and treatment of the different pathologies of the temporomandibular joint. The reconstructive procedures must carefully assess all these factors to achieve long-term success. The purpose of this chapter is to analyze the temporomandibular joint encompassing anatomy, physiology with a biomechanical approach for its diagnosis and treatment.

Keywords: temporomandibular joint, temporomandibular biomechanics, temporomandibular anatomy, temporomandibular physiology

1. Introduction

The temporomandibular joint (TMJ) can be classified by its function and by its anatomy. Functionally it is ginglymoarthrodial, a term derived from ginglymus, meaning a hinge joint, allowing movement only forwards and backwards in one plane, and arthrodial, meaning a joint allowing sliding movement of surfaces [1]. Anatomically, it is a diarthrodial joint, defined as the discontinuous articulation of two bones that allow freedom of movement. The movement of the TMJ is dictated by muscles and limited by ligaments, its capsule of fibrous connective tissue is innervated, vascularized and strongly attached to the joint surfaces. It is also a synovial joint, whose fluid acts as a joint lubricant and supplies its metabolic and nutritional needs [2]. When occluding the mandible, it will be subjected to loads, a unilateral occlusion will result in load peaks at the contralateral TMJ. In addition, the condyle is an adaptable and regenerative unit with the ability to maintain functions despite trauma and degenerative changes [3]. The TMJ is the only joint in the human body that houses a growth center, resulting in the perpetual need for the left and right joints to work coordinated [4].

Biomechanics is the study of mechanics applied to living beings, it analyzes loads, efforts, tension, movement, size, shape and structure of the body. The temporomandibular joint is subject to forces produced by the masticatory muscles and the occlusion stress that is supported by the teeth [3]. In addition, it analyzes and helps understand the interaction of form, function and mechanism of the temporomandibular disorders to prevent, diagnose and cure these disorders [5]. A total joint replacement should function as close to a healthy joint as possible. It must be able to withstand the same forces and must produce the same movements as a normal joint [6].

2. Components of the temporomandibular joint

2.1 Temporary component

The temporal bone contributes three regions to the TMJ, the largest being the articular or mandibular fossa, a concave surface whose anterior limit is the articular eminence, and its posterior limit is the postglenoid process [2]. The glenoid fossa is wider mediolaterally than anteroposteriorly, its surface is thin, and it may be translucent in a dissected skull, showing that although the articular fossa contains the posterior edge of the disc and condyle, it's not a functionally resistant tension part [1, 7]. The second portion, the articular eminence, is a transverse bony prominence that continues mediolaterally across the articular surface, is generally thick, and serves as a major functional component of the TMJ. The third portion of the articular surface of the temporal bone is the preglenoid plane, a flattened area anterior to the eminence [2, 7].

2.2 Mandibular component

The mandibular portion that is part of the TMJ is the condyle, it's a paired structure that forms an angle of approximately 145° to 160° with each other. It normally has an elliptical shape and measures on average 20 mm mediolaterally (range 13 to 25 mm) and 10 mm anteroposteriorly (range 5.5 to 16 mm). The condyle tends to be rounded mediolaterally and convex anteroposteriorly. The size and shape of the condyle present large individual variations that may be relevant in terms of biomechanical load. In its medial portion below its articular surface is the pterygoid fovea, site of insertions of the lateral pterygoid muscle [2, 8].

2.3 Cartilage and synovium

Lining the inner face of the joint, there are two types of tissue: articular and synovial cartilage. The space bounded by these two structures is called the synovial cavity, which is filled with synovial fluid. The articular surfaces of the temporal bone and condyle are covered with dense articular fibrocartilage. This cover has the ability to regenerate and remodel under functional stress. Deep to the fibrocartilage of the condyle, there is a proliferative zone of cells that can become cartilage or bone tissue. Articular cartilage is composed of chondrocytes and an intercellular matrix of collagen fibers, water, and a nonfibrous tissue, filling material, called the ground substance. Chondrocytes are arranged in three layers characterized by different cell shapes. The superficial zone contains small flattened cells with their longitudinal axes parallel to the surface. In the middle zone the cells are larger and rounder and appear in columns perpendicular to the surface. The deep zone contains the largest cells and is divided by the Level mark; below which some degree of calcification occurs [2].

Cartilage is nourished primarily by diffusion from synovial fluid. Collagen fibers are arranged in an interlocking meshwork of fibrils parallel to the joint surface, joining as bundles and descending to them junction in the calcified cartilage between the level marks. Functionally, these meshes provide a framework for the interstitial water and the essential substance to resist the compressive forces encountered in the load [2].

Articular cartilage contains a higher proportion of collagen fibers than other synovial joints. The fundamental substance contains a variety of plasma proteins, glucose, urea and salts, as well as proteoglycans, which are synthesized by the Golgi apparatus of chondrocytes. Proteoglycans are macromolecules that contain a protein core linked to chondroitin sulfate and keratan sulfate glycosaminoglycan chains. Proteoglycans are involved in the diffusion of nutrients and metabolic degradation. The ground substance allows the entry and exit of large amounts of water, allowing its characteristic functional elasticity in response to deformation and load [2, 8].

The lining of the capsule is the synovial membrane, a thin, smooth, richly vascular, and innervated membrane that contains no epithelium. Synovial cells have a phagocytic and secretory function and are believed to be the site of hyaluronic acid production. Synovial fluid is considered an ultrafiltrate of plasma which comes from two sources: the first, from plasma by dialysis, and the second, from the secretion of type A and B synoviocytes [1, 2]. Among its functions is the lubrication of the joint, phagocytosis of particles and nutrition of the articular cartilage. It contains a high concentration of hyaluronic acid. The proteins found in synovial fluid are identical to plasma proteins; however, it has a lower total protein content, a higher percentage of albumin, and a lower percentage of α −2-globulin.

The number of leukocytes is less than 200 per cubic millimeter and less than 25% of these cells are polymorphonuclear. Only a small amount of synovial fluid, usually less than 2 ml, is present within the healthy TMJ [2].

2.4 The articular disc

Its biconcave in shape with a length of approximately 12 mm and a width of 16 mm. It is firmly attached to the lateral and medial poles of the condyle [9]. made up of dense fibrous connective tissue and is not vascularized or innervated, an adaptation that allows it to resist pressure, is composed of densely organized collagen fibers, high molecular weight proteoglycans, elastic fibers, and cells ranging from fibrocytes to chondrocytes. Collagen is mainly made up of types I and II. The fibers have a typical pattern of distribution in the intermediate zone, oriented sagittally and parallel to the disc surface. Most of these fibers continue into the anterior and posterior bands to intertwine or continue with the oriented collagen fibers transversely and vertically of these bands or pass through the entire bands to continue towards the anterior and posterior disc attachments. Vertically and transversely oriented fibers are more pronounced in the anterior and posterior band. In the intermediate part there is weaker cross-linking of the collagen bundles, which makes this area less resistant to mediolateral shear stresses [8].

Anatomically the disc can be divided into three regions in a sagittal section: an anterior portion (about 2 mm), posterior portion (about 3 mm), and a middle portion of 1 mm. The anterior portion of the disc consists of a layer of fibroelastic fascia (upper) and a fibrous layer (lower). The disc is flexible and adapts to the demands of the joint surfaces, joining the capsule anteriorly, posteriorly, medially, and laterally [2, 7]. It's bounded inferiorly by the articular surface of the mandibular condyle and laterally and medially by the synovial membrane. It divides the inferior and superior joint compartment into two spaces. The inferior joint space contains approximately 0.9 ml of synovial fluid, while the superior joint space contains approximately 1.2 ml [9].

Articular disc has been shown to have region- and direction-dependent variations in biomechanical response. Female joint discs tend to be stiffer and relax less than male discs, suggesting a possible etiologic factor in the development and progression of temporomandibular disorders, and the higher prevalence among women [10].

The presence of a fibrocartilaginous disc in the joint prevents peak loads because it has the capacity to deform and adapt to the joint surfaces. These deformations ensure that the loads are absorbed and distributed over larger contact areas. In addition, the shape of the disc and the location of the contact zones continuously change during mandibular movement to adapt to the articulating surfaces. As a result, there will be a change in the magnitude and location of the deformations [11].

2.5 Retrodiscal tissue

The retrodiscal area is called the bilaminar zone because it consists of two laminae separated by loose connective tissue made up of elastic fibers, blood vessels, lymphatics, nerves, and adipose tissue. The inferior lamina inserts into the periosteum of the condyle approximately 8 to 10 mm below the condylar apex. The lamina consists of thick fibers that originate from almost the entire height of the posterior band and lacks elastic fibers. The lamina stretches with occlusion and bends as the condyle rotates into the mandibular opening. It is believed to serve as a control ligament to prevent extreme rotation of the disc at the condyle in rotational movements [2, 8]. On the other hand, the upper lamina inserts into the periosteum of the fossa anterior to the squamotympanic and petrotympanic fissures, is thinner than the lower lamina and contains thinner collagen fibers. It has elastic fibers and collagen fibers that fold in the occluded position and stretch during opening or protrusion, allowing the disc to slide anteriorly. The position of the disc is ensured by the lateral and posterior inferior ligaments [8].

The loose tissue of the retrocondylar space compensates for pressure changes that arise when the retrocondylar space expands during translation. The loose fibroelastic structure allows the blood vessels to expand, causing the posterior superior lamina to press against the fossa and the posterior inferior lamina to fold superiorly. The blood vessels are connected with the pterygoid venous plexus located anteromedially to the condyle. Therefore, during opening, blood drains backwards and laterally to fill the enlarged space behind the condyle, and upon closing, it is pushed into the pterygoid plexus [8].

2.6 Ligaments

They are composed of collagen and act predominantly as restraints on movement of the condyle and disc. Three ligaments can be considered main: collateral, capsular and temporomandibular ligaments. Other ligaments such as the sphenomandibular, stylomandibular, pterygomandibular, and Pinto ligaments are considered accessory ligaments because they serve to some extent as passive restrictors in mandibular movement [2, 7].

2.6.1 Collateral or discal ligaments

They are short paired structures that span each joint, they attach superiorly to the temporal bone along the rim of the glenoid fossa and articular eminence, and inferiorly to the neck of the condyle along the rim of the articular facet. It surrounds the joint spaces and the disc, being attached anteriorly and posteriorly, as well as medially and laterally. The function is to resist medial, lateral and inferior forces, thus maintaining the attachment of the disc to the condyle. This offers protection in extreme movements, a secondary function is to contain the synovial fluid within the superior and inferior joint spaces [2, 7].

2.6.2 Temporomandibular (lateral) ligaments

They are found on the lateral aspect of each TMJ or temporomandibular joint. They are individual structures that function in pairs with the corresponding ligament in the opposite TMJ. It can be separated into two different parts, which have different functions. The external oblique part descends from the external aspect of the articular tubercle of the zygomatic process and inferiorly to the external posterior surface of the condylar neck. It limits the amount of inferior distraction that the condyle can have in translation and rotation movements. The internal horizontal part also arises from the external surface of the articular tubercle, just medial to the origin of the external oblique part of the ligament, and runs horizontally posteriorly to join the lateral pole of the condyle and the posterior pole of the disc. The function of the inner portion is to limit the posterior movement of the condyle, particularly during rotational movements, for example when the mandible moves laterally in masticatory function [2, 7].

2.6.3 Sphenomandibular ligament

It is a remnant of Merckel's cartilage. It originates from the sphenoid spine and on its way to the mandible inserts into the medial wall of the TMJ joint capsule. It continues its descent to attach to the lingula of the mandible as well as to the lower part of the medial side of the condylar neck. Its main function is to protect the TMJ of an excessive translation of the condyle, after 10 degrees of opening of the mouth, also functions as a point of rotation during the activation of the lateral pterygoid muscle [2, 7].

2.6.4 Stylomandibular ligament

The stylomandibular ligament arises from the styloid process to the posterior margin of the mandible or the angle of the mandible. It is considered a thickening of the deep cervical fascia. Its function is to limit the excessive protrusion of the mandible [2, 7].

2.6.5 Pterygomandibular ligament

The pterygomandibular ligament or raphe (PTML) is a thickening of the oropharyngeal fascia. It arises from the apex of the hamulus of the internal pterygoid plane of the skull to the posterior zone of the retromolar trigone of the mandible, limiting its movements [2, 7].

2.6.6 Pinto or malleomandibular or discomalleolar ligament

It has two parts: The first part refers to the middle ear involving the malleus in relation to the anterior ligament of the malleus; the second, the portion of the joint capsule of the TMJ, in contact with the retrodiscal tissues. The functions are two. In the TMJ it protects the synovial membrane with respect to the tensions of the structures surrounding and in the middle ear, would seem to control or influence the appropriate pressure for this area of the ear [2, 7].

3. Irrigation

The vascular supply of the TMJ arises mainly from branches of the superficial temporal artery, the maxillary artery, and the masseteric artery. All arteries within a radius of 3 cm contribute to the vascularization of the TMJ through the appearance of secondary capillaries that branch to surround the joint capsule [12]. Venous drainage occurs through the pterygoid plexus in the retrodiscal area, which alternately fills and empties in protrusion and retrusion movements, respectively, to subsequently communicate with the internal maxillary vein, the sphenopalatine vein, the medial meningeal veins, the deep temporal veins, the masseteric veins and the inferior alveolar vein [7].

Lymphatic drainage is not always easy to describe because, in the case of TMJ disease, the lymph nodes may increase in number. Generally, the lymphatic system that drains the TMJ comes from the area of the submandibular triangle [7].

4. Innervation

The TMJ has several proprioceptive receptors, particularly in the parenchyma of the articular disc: Golgi—Mazzoni and Ruffini; Myelinated and unmyelinated nerve fibers are innervated primarily by the auriculotemporal nerve posteriorly, the masseteric nerve anteriorly, the posterior deep temporal nerve anteromedially, and the branch of the TMJ arising directly from the mandibular nerve anteriorly. The middle part, although there are variations in these innervation pathways [13].

5. Muscles

Classically, four masticatory muscles are described: temporal, masseter, lateral and medial pterygoid, although the supra and infrahyoid muscles also participate in mandibular movements [14].

5.1 Temporal muscle

The function of the temporalis muscle is to elevate the mandible for closure. It is not a power muscle. Contractions of the middle and posterior portions of the muscle contribute to retrusion of the mandible, and a small degree of unilateral contraction of the temporal bone assists in deviation of the mandible to the ipsilateral side [14].

5.2 Masseter muscle

Both the superficial and deep parts of the masseter muscle are powerful elevators of the jaw, but they function independently and reciprocally in some movements.

The deep layer of the masseter is not active during protrusive movements and is always active during forced retrusion, whereas the superficial portion is active during protrusion and is inactive during retrusion. Similarly, the deep masseter is active in ipsilateral movements but does not function in contralateral movements, while the superficial masseter is active during contralateral movements but not in ipsilateral movements [14].

5.3 Medial pterygoid muscle

The primary function of the medial pterygoid is elevation of the mandible, but it also has a limited role in unilateral protrusion in synergism with the lateral pterygoid to promote rotation to the opposite side [14].

5.4 Lateral pterygoid muscle

It has two portions that can be considered two functionally distinct muscles. The main function of the lower head is protrusive and contralateral movement. When the two inferior bundles contract, the condyle is pulled forward and below the articular eminence, with the disc moving passively with the condylar head. This movement contributes to the opening of the oral cavity. When the inferior head works unilaterally, it produces a contralateral movement of the mandible. The function of the superior bundles is predominantly involved with the closing and retrusion movements [14].

5.5 Supra and infrahyoid muscles

This group of muscles is formed by 4 suprahyoid pairs that are digastric, mylohyoid, stylohyoid and geniohyoid and 4 infrahyoid pairs that are sternohyoid, omohyoid, sternothyroid and thyrohyoid whose function in mandibular movements is to fix or move the hyoid [14].

6. Mandibular movements and muscle activity

Mandibular movement during function and parafunction involves complex neuromuscular patterns originating and modifying from central and peripheral origin. The ATM contributes about 2000 movements per day [11, 15].

6.1 Jaw opening

The active muscles are the digastric, mylohyoid, and geniohyoid. There is no activity in the temporal when there is a slow opening and the mandible is in maximum opening, although some activity can occur in the medial pterygoid [15].

6.2 Jaw closure

There is no temporary activity during mandibular closure as long as there is no contact with the teeth. The elevation without contact is given by the masseter and medial pterygoid [15].

6.3 Retrusion

Voluntary retrusion in mandibular closure is given by the contraction of the posterior fibers of the temporalis muscle, as well as by the suprahyoid and infrahoid muscle groups [15].

6.4 Protrusion

Protrusion without occlusal contact is the result of contraction of the lateral and medial pterygoids as well as the bilateral masseters [15].

6.5 Lateral movements

Lateral movement of the mandible without tooth contact is achieved primarily by contraction of the medial and posterior fibers of the ipsilateral temporalis muscle and by contralateral contraction of the lateral and medial pterygoid and anterior temporalis fibers. The suprahyoid muscles are active keeping the mandible slightly protruded and depressed [15].

7. Mandibular kinematics

Functionally, mandibular movements are complex with six degrees of possible movement, which occur as complex interrelated rotational and translational activities. They are possible thanks to the relationship of four different joints: lower and upper. Although the TMJ does not function independently of the other, a classification of isolated mandibular movements is necessary [11, 16].

7.1 Types of movements

Movements have been extensively studied at the level of the occlusal interface, being Ulf Posselt one of the first to describe motion in three dimensions. Condylar rotation and translation of the condyle-disc assembly, in most cases, begin simultaneously. On average, condylar rotation increases or decreases linearly by approximately 2°/mm of anterior or posterior translation during opening or closing, respectively [8, 16].

7.2 Rotational movement

Rotation occurs when the condyles rotate around a fixed point or axis during mandibular opening and closing. Rotational motion can occur in three reference planes: horizontal, vertical, and sagittal. Each of them occurs around a point called the axis [11].

- Horizontal orientation axis: opening and closing movement, referred to as a hinge, therefore it occurs around an axis called the hinge axis. It is considered the purest rotation movement [16].

- Vertical axis of rotation: Also called frontal axis. It occurs when one of the condyles moves anteriorly from the position of the terminal hinge axis with the vertical axis in the opposite condyle, which remains in said axis. This type of movement does not occur normally [16].

- Sagittal axis of rotation: Occurs when one of the condyles moves inferiorly while the other remains in the position of the terminal axis. This movement occurs in conjunction with other movements. Mathematical studies indicate that in this plane there is the same contact and muscle activity from one side to the other, so there are no alterations in dental occlusion that result in a joint without load [11, 16].

The amount of condylar rotation does not differ between men and women. A finding that contrasts with the greater maximum interincisal opening of men compared to women due to differences in jaw length. In fact, with the same degree of rotation, the greater the length of the mandible, the greater the opening of the mouth. Consequently, the degree of interincisal opening cannot be considered as a measure of joint mobility or laxity, unless corrected for mandibular size [8].

7.3 Translational motion

Translation can be defined as a movement in which every point of the object t simultaneously has the same speed and direction. In the masticatory system, it occurs when the mandible protrudes. During normal movements, rotation and translation occur simultaneously, as the mandible rotates in one or more axes, each of the axes is changing orientation in space [16].

The total movement of the mandible does not consist only of rotation and translation. Side-to-side or eccentric bodily movement of the mandible and rotation and translation of the joints indicate that the mandible acts as a free-moving or floating; structure. Controlled by pairs of complementary and opposing functional muscle groups that gradually exert impulse force with numerous force vectors, the three-dimensional movement of the mandible with a dual-operation joint system is unlike any other orthopedic system in the body [17].

Classical records analyzed mandibular movements in terms of their geometry, using mechanical systems. Posselt designed an instrument called a gnatho-tensiometer, which could record border movements in all three planes, obtaining the Posselt diagram. Currently, technology has made it possible to improve position tracking techniques and thus be able to analyze mandibular kinematics with high spatial and temporal resolution (**Figure 1**) [18].

7.4 Temporomandibular joint and its relationship with occlusion

Movement is not only guided by the shape of the bones, muscles, and ligaments, but also by the occlusion of the teeth [1]. The Glossary of Prosthodontic Terms defines occlusion as the static relationship between the chewing surfaces of the maxillary and mandibular teeth. Dental contact has to be studied from a functional perspective and a more adequate definition of occlusion would be the biological and dynamic relationship of the components of the masticatory system that determines dental relationships [19].

Occlusion comprises a wide range of topics, the biomechanics of occlusal contact between two teeth with different cusp inclinations form a complex system [16]. From a clinical point of view, TMJ changes including intracapsular exudate and joint tissue

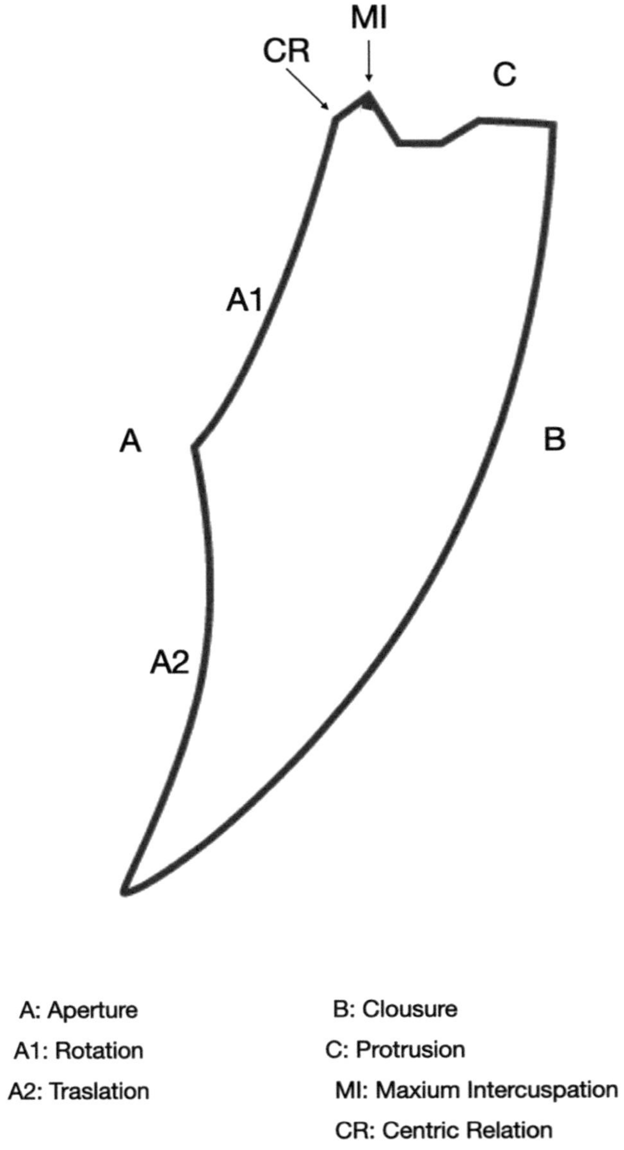

Figure 1.
Posselt diagram.

loss can result in occlusal changes such as anterior or posterior open bites. It is important to mention that a particular occlusal scheme is not a determinant of disease. There is no evidence to suggest that one scheme predominates over another. Group functions compared to canine guides cause less condylar displacement, this displacement is small and has no clinical significance [19].

The range of vertical movement is dictated by anterior determinants such as overbite and posterior determinants such as TMJ condylar guidance. From a biomechanical point of view, anterior versus posterior determinants have a greater influence on tooth contact due to their proximity to the teeth. On the other hand, the condylar guide will influence when the molars are in contact or close to contact during mandibular movements [19].

7.5 Loads at the TMJ

Studies about whether the TMJ is subjected to load has been the subject of discussion for many years. Brehnan et al. in 1981 was able to corroborate in his studies carried out on monkeys that there is a load in the TMJ. It's accepted that mechanical loading is essential for growth [11]. During the natural function of the joint, a combination of compressive, tensile, and shear loads occur [5]. The efforts produced by the loads will generate a deformation which can be quantified by determining the change between the original length with the final length of a structure, this deformation is expressed as a percentage, there are two types of deformation: elastic

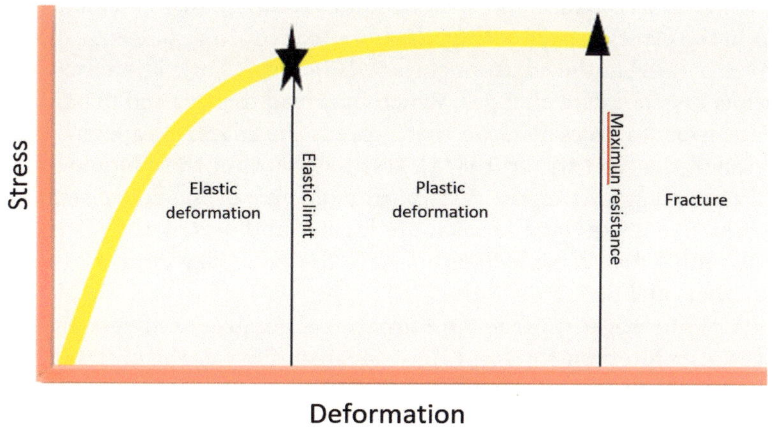

Figure 2.
Graph shows that the elastic limit and the maximun resistance.

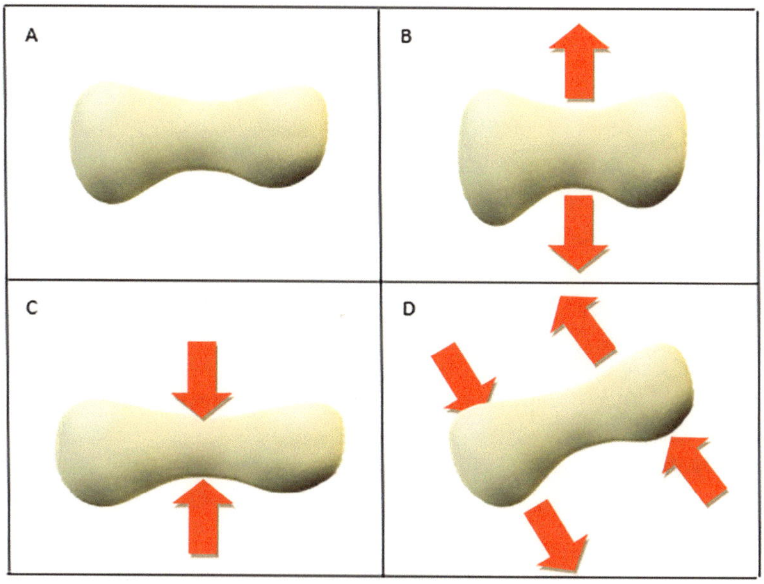

Figure 3.
Different types of load over disc. A. Normal state. B. Tension. C. Compression D. shear.

one in which eliminating the force the material recovers its original dimension, while plastic deformation is one in which the original dimension is not recovered. The elastic limit es the yield point beyond which permanent deformation occurs and the tissue does not return to its original shape. Ultimate strength is the stress a tissue can withstand, and breaking strength is the stress at which the tissue breaks (**Figure 2**) [20].

The value of the maximum resistance of the disc depends on the direction of the applied stress and the region where it is applied. For example, the ultimate strength of the intermediate zone of the disc is 37.4 MPa (1 MPa = 106N/m2) when a tensile stress is applied anteroposteriorly, while it is 1.6 MPa when the application of stress is medio-lateral [11].

During compressive loading the disk becomes smaller, during tensile loading, it is stretched in the direction of loading, during shear loading, one edge of the disk surface moves parallel to the adjacent surface (**Figure 3**) [16]. Therefore, an unloaded TMJ may show degenerative changes, which may lead to impaired masticatory function. However, an excessive load that exceeds the adaptive capacity can also lead to degradation of the joint structure [11]. If the surfaces of the condyle or fossa have significant bony irregularities, the distribution of force over an even smaller square area of the joint can make these ratios more diverse and destructive. Otherwise, an aging dysfunctional disc/capsule does not have the necessary viscoelastic properties to meet the functional demands of the TMJ [17].

Any surgical procedure must restore functional congruence between all four joint surfaces. Any intervention must limit the instability of the joint to eliminate the progressive influence of torque and shear at the lateral attachment of the disc/capsule to the mandibular condyle. Currently, no synthetic or biological material meets the viscoelastic properties disk/capsule Knowledge of biomechanics will guide the clinician in making decisions for the surgical treatment of TMJ.

Author details

Pablo Andrés Crespo Reinoso[1]*, Emilio Ruiz Delgado[2] and James Jerez Robalino[3]

1 Oral and Maxillofacial Surgery. Private practice

2 Department of Prosthodontics and Implantology, Universidad de Cuenca, Ecuador

3 Faculty of Dentistry, Universidad Nacional Autónoma de México, Resident Department of Oral and Maxillofacial Surgery, Ciudad Universitaria, México

*Address all correspondence to: pablocrespood@gmail.com

References

[1] Alomar X, Medrano J, Cabratosa J, Clavero J, Lorente M, Serra I, et al. Anatomy of the temporomandibular joint. Seminars in Ultrasound, CT and MRI. 2007;**28**(3):170-183. DOI: 10.1053/j.sult.2007.02.002

[2] Miloro M, Larsen PE, Ghali GE, Waite PD. Peterson's Principles of Oral and Maxillofacial Surgery. Second ed. Hamilton (Canada) and London (UK): B. C. Decker, Inc; 2004. p. 1502

[3] Roberts WE, Goodacre CJ. The temporomandibular joint: A critical review of life-support functions, development, articular surfaces. Biomechanics and Degeneration. J Prosthodont. 2020;**29**(9):772-779. DOI: 10.1111/jopr.13203

[4] Stanković S, Vlajković S, Bošković M, Radenković G, Antić V, Jevremović D. Morphological and biomechanical features of the temporomandibular joint disc: An overview of recent findings. Archives of Oral Biology. 2013;**58**(10):1475-1482. DOI: 10.1016/j.archoralbio.2013.06.014

[5] Ingawale S. Temporomandibular joint: Disorders, treatments and biomechanics. Annals of Biomedical Engineering. 2009;**37**(5):976-996

[6] Gaylord S. Throckmorton, temporomandibular joint biomechanics. Oral and Maxillofacial Surgery Clinics of North America. 2000;**12**(1):27-42. DOI: 10.1016/S1042-3699(20)30229-6

[7] Bordoni B, Varacallo M. Anatomy, head and neck, temporomandibular joint. In: StatPearls. Treasure Island (FL): StatPearls Publishing; 2022. Available from: https://www.ncbi.nlm.nih.gov/books/NBK538486/

[8] Palla S. Chapter 6—Anatomy and pathophysiology of the temporomandibular joint. In: Klineberg I, Eckert SE, editors. Functional Occlusion in Restorative Dentistry and Prosthodontics. United States; 2016. pp. 67-85. DOI: 10.1016/B978-0-7234-3809-0.00006-1

[9] González-García R, Gil-Díez Usandizaga JL, Rodríguez-Campo FJ. Arthroscopic anatomy and lysis and lavage of the temporomandibular joint. Atlas of the Oral and Maxillofacial Surgery Clinics of North America. 2011;**19**(2):131-144. DOI: 10.1016/j.cxom.2011.05.002

[10] Wright GJ, Coombs MC, Hepfer RG, Damon BJ, Bacro TH, Lecholop MK, et al. Tensile biomechanical properties of human temporomandibular joint disc: Effects of direction, region and sex. Journal of Biomechanics. 2016;**49**(16):3762-3769. DOI: 10.1016/j.jbiomech.2016.09.033

[11] Tanaka E. Biomechanical behavior of the temporomandibular joint disc. Critical Reviews in Oral Biology & Medicine. 2003;**14**(2):138-150

[12] Faustino D, Nogueira J, Pinheiro C, Alves G, Cardoso H. Temporomandibular joint arterial variability. Journal of Cranio-Maxillofacial Surgery. 2021. DOI: 10.1016/j.jcms.2021.12.006 Feb;**50**(2):150-155

[13] Kucukguven A, Demiryurek MD, Vargel I. Temporomandibular joint innervation: Anatomical study and clinical implications. Annals of Anatomy. 2022;**240**:151882. DOI: 10.1016/j.aanat.2021.151882

[14] Rouvière H, Delmas A. Human Anatomy Descriptive, Topographical and Functional. Masson. Ed. 11ª. 2005

[15] Nelson ST, Ash MM. Wheeler's Dental Anatomy, Physiology and Occlusion. 9th ed. Philadelphia, PA: WB Saunders Co; 2010

[16] Okeson J. Managment of Temporomandibular Disorders and Occlusion. United States; 2020

[17] Kirk WS Jr, Kirk BS. A biomechanical basis for primary arthroplasty of the temporomandibular joint. Oral and Maxillofacial Surgery Clinics of North America. 2006;**18**(3):345-368. DOI: 10.1016/j.coms.2006.03.006

[18] Vargas S. Analisis tridimensional de movimientos mandibulares bordeantes en participantes dentados totales. International Journal of Morphology. 2020;**38**(4):983-989

[19] Peck C. Biomechanics of occlusion—Implications for oral rehabilitation. Journal of Oral Rehabilitation. 2016;**45**:205-214

[20] Crespo P, Jerez J, González de Santiago M. Biomechanics of midface trauma: A review of concepts. Journal of Oral and Maxillofacial Surgery, Medicine, and Pathology. 2021;**33**(4):389-393. DOI: 10.1016/j.ajoms.2021.01.010

Chapter 6

Exploring the Association between Temporomandibular Joint Disorder (TMD) and Orthodontics

Siddharth Mehta

Abstract

Temporomandibular joint is an important bilateral synovial joint of body. This chapter focuses on the basic anatomy of TMJ and its disorders. Any pain or symptom of TMJ falls under the category of temporomandibular joint disorder. There is a decade old debate of cause-effect relationship of malocclusion and temporomandibular joint disorder. How orthodontic treatment can positively contribute to this problem is highlighted in this chapter.

Keywords: temporomandibular joint disorder, orthodontics, malocclusion, anatomy

1. Introduction

The temporomandibular joint is the joint that joins lower jaw (mandible) to the skull. It is a bilateral synovial joint formed between the articular surface of temporal bone and condylar head of the mandible. The functioning of the joint is together and not independent of the other. The main components of the joint are the capsule, disc, articular surface of temporal bone, temporomandibular ligament, stylomandibular ligament, sphenomandibular ligament, and lateral pterygoid muscle [1].

The articular capsule (capsular ligament) is a thin loose envelope, attached above to the mandibular fossa and the articular tubercle below. The disc is a dense fibrocartilage positioned between the mandibular fossa and the articular surface of the head of condyle. This synovial joint is divided into two compartments by the disc *viz.* upper and lower joint compartment. Capsule's synovial membrane fills these compartments with synovial fluid and provides lubrication. The central area of the disc is avascular with no innervation, and synovial fluid nourishes the disc. The posterior ligament and the surrounding capsule have both blood vessels and innervation. The central area is thinner and of denser consistency; peripheral is thicker and cushioned. Age-related changes may thin the disc and add cartilage to the center and may lead to impaired movement of the joint. Disc is a fibrous extension of the capsule between the two bones, and is biconcave and attached to the condyle medially and laterally. Anterior portion of the disc divides backward vertically and continues as retrodiscal tissue; forwardly, the split becomes coincident with the superior head of lateral pterygoid. The lower joint compartment allows the rotational movement, while opening and upper joint compartment allows translation.

TMJ has three ligaments: one major and two minor ligaments. Ligaments define the extent of movement of mandible. If movements go beyond the extent allowed by muscles, pain will arise. Major ligament, the temporomandibular ligament is in reality, thickened lateral portion of the capsule. It has two parts: an outer oblique and an inner horizontal portion. This ligament is shaped like a triangle with base attaching to the zygomatic process of temporal bone and articular tubercle, and apex at lateral side of the neck of the mandible. This ligament prevents the retraction/distal movement of the mandible and thus protects the joint. The rest of the minor ligaments sphenomandibular and stylomandibular ligaments are not attached to the joint. Stylomandibular ligament runs from the styloid process to the angle of the mandible and becomes tight on mandibular protrusion. Sphenomandibular ligament, a remnant of Meckel's cartilage, runs from the spine of sphenoid to the lingula of mandible, which also becomes tight with mandibular protrusion. Other ligaments are otomandibular, discomallear, and malleomandibular ligament.

Blood supply: Superficial temporal branch of external carotid artery majorly innervates the joint.

Nerve supply: Auriculotemporal and masseteric branches of mandibular branch of trigeminal nerve provide sensory innervation to the TMJ. Proprioreception occurs through four receptors: Ruffini endings, Golgi tendon organs (static), Pacinian corpuscles (dynamic), and free nerve endings (pain). Free nerve endings are present in the bones, ligaments, and muscles except the fibrocartilage).

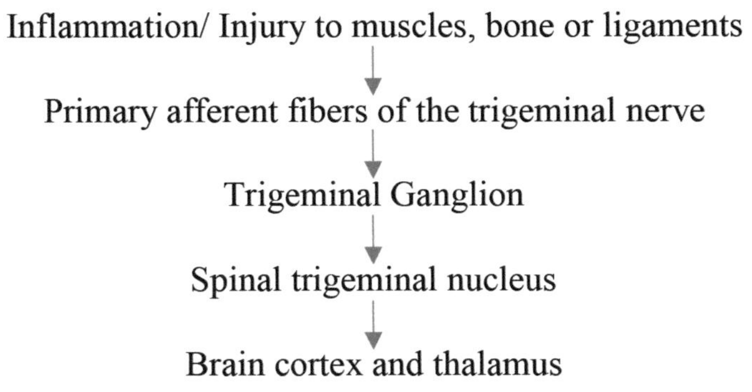

2. Temporomandibular dysfunction (TMD)

TMD is a term involving dysfunction and pain of the masticatory muscles, joint, and surrounding tissues. It is one of the most common cause of facial pain, which is non-dental in origin [2–4].

Signs and symptoms of TMD:

1. Headache.

2. Pain behind eyes.

3. Ear pain with no infection.

4. Discomfort and limited mouth opening.

5. Bruxism/tooth grinding at night.

6. Localized/generalized sensitivity of teeth.

7. Wear facets.

8. Clicking sounds.

9. Joint tenderness/muscle tenderness.

10. Neck stiffness.

11. Swallowing difficulties.

12. Sore throat with no infection.

2.1 Prevalence

In a systematic review published by Lai et al. in 2020, it was reported that prevalence of TMD ranges from 21.1 to 73.3%. About 3.4–65.7% of patients reported pain as TMD signs and symptoms and non-painful ranged from 3.1 to 40.8%. The study showed greater predilection of TMD for females than males and adults (>18 years) than young patients. Though this study reported no correlation of malocclusion to TMD, there are implications of several occlusal traits.

2.2 Temporomandibular dysfunction (TMD) and malocclusion

Relationship of occlusion with TMDs has long been debated. Costen's syndrome as given by Dr. James Costen correlated TMJ pain, headache, limited mandibular opening, and ear symptoms with increased overbite. Thompson suggested correction of malocclusion to correct TMJ symptoms.

Malocclusion, be it skeletal or dental, shows disharmony in all the three planes of space—sagittal, vertical, and transverse.

2.2.1 Transverse malocclusions

Unilateral posterior cross-bite is found to be mostly related to TMJ clicking and myofascial pain. It is thought that patients with such a situation have abnormal contacts that affect the relationship between condyle and fossa. Case studies have shown that improving the occlusal factors by orthodontic treatment did not completely improve the TMD symptoms reflective of anatomic contribution of glenoid fossa and condyle head. Through electro-myographic studies, it was concluded that unilateral posterior cross-bite causes asymmetric activation of masticatory muscles leading to overloading on one side and joint symptoms. Though symptoms were more commonly observed in adults than in growing patients, surveys have shown role of emotional well-being and sleep bruxism on TMD symptoms. A recent study by Yap et al. reported a higher level of psychological disturbance and poor quality of life in patients with moderate-to-severe TMD [5, 6]. Acupuncture has been shown to be effective in reducing pain and improving quality of life in TMD patients [7].

2.2.2 Sagittal and vertical malocclusions

Evidence shows correlation between TMD and increased overjet, vertical growth patterns, open bite malocclusions, disc displacements and degenerative changes.

To sum up, TMDs have a multifactorial etiology and cause effect relationship between occlusion and disorders have to be further explored as some occlusal changes may be the result rather than a cause of malocclusion.

2.3 Temporomandibular disorders (TMDs) and orthodontics

Clinical management of TMDs has been a topic of controversy for nearly 100 years. There have been two events in the history that have attracted attention of the dental fields. The first was in 1934 when Costen related TMJ and ear pain to changes in the vertical dimension. Second was Gnathological society papers that correlated balance between functioning of the jaw and occlusal positions. The aim was to achieve a canine protected occlusion and no centric relation-centric occlusion (CR-CO) discrepancy [2].

Since then, various theories have been formulated to understand TMDs. Orthodontic Stalwarts like Brodie, Moyers, Ricketts have worked significantly to understand the concept of TMJ, Jaw function, and occlusion. Ronald Roth played an important role in introducing the concept of gnathology and prosthodontics into orthodontic patients. He suggested optimal functional occlusal goals by coinciding CR with CO. To achieve these goals, he suggested Roth power bite registration and use of articulators. These philosophies were in contrast to another group of orthodontists who were against traditional premolar extraction in orthodontics and retainer wear and attributed TMDs to extraction.

Interesting turn of events happened in 1987 in Brimm vs. Malloy Michigan lawsuit in which a 16-year-old female was treated for a class 2 malocclusion with a 7-mm overjet with upper first premolar extraction, fixed orthodontics, and headgear. After removal of fixed appliances, during retainer wear, she complained of headache and joint pain. She had no signs of TMD before or during the treatment. She was referred to an oral surgeon for removal of lower third molar. This further increased her problem as she developed severe pain, clicking, and locking of joint.

Following lawsuit, Oral surgeon was sued for $2500 for not being able to diagnose TMD and Orthodontist was sued for $85,000 for causing internal derangement of TMJ by extraction and over-retraction of incisors resulting in distal displacement of mandible.

In 1992, January issue of AJODO, studies done by American Association of Orthodontists were published concluding no association between jaw structure and TMDs. It also stated that the development of TMDs cannot be predicted. TMD symptoms may increase with age; thus, TMD symptoms may arise during orthodontic treatment but may not be related to treatment. TMD correction may not be assured once present, though evidence supports the beneficial effect of orthodontics in reducing the symptoms of TMD.

3. What do we know till now?

Based on evidence accumulated over years, it is supported that orthodontic treatment with or without exodontia, head gear use, chin cup, elastics or deep bite correction do not cause TMDs and upper incisors can be safely retracted. This does not cause distal position of condyles and consequent anterior position of the disk.

Best way to plan treatment is in patients with original jaw relation in centric occlusion and no dual bite present. Patients' condyle position should be protected throughout fixed orthodontic and adjunctive treatment, and any procedure that may shift the condyles away from the original physiologic position may affect the patient.

Clinical Trials by OPPERA (Orofacial Pain: Prospective evaluation and risk assessment trials) have shifted emphasis of TMDs from a mechanical to a biopsychological mode of management. Placebo medications, deprogramming appliance therapy, and occlusal equilibration only have yielded favorable responses, and it becomes clear that there may be another pathway to alleviate pain and shifting to invasive, and more aggressive treatments should be deferred if conservative and reversible TMJ treatments are possible [2, 8–11].

4. What can be the contribution of orthodontists?

1. Develop an evidence based clinical practice.

2. Conduct a proper TMJ examination and educating the patient about appearance of symptoms during or after treatment if predisposing factors exist.

3. Document all findings and informed consent.

4. Address TMJ pain before starting orthodontic therapy.

5. Avoid diagnosis and treating TMDs within mechanical boundaries. If symptoms arise during the active treatment phase, stop all the treatments and focus on managing TMJ pain. Try to manage with conservative and reversible methods.

5. Do's for TMD patients

1. Biopsychosocial profile modulation by the patient has shown to be beneficial.

2. Fruit and vegetable diet is helpful to reduce the pain.

3. Use of cannabidiol oils help reduce anxiety.

4. Craniosacral therapy—Gentle fascia palpation techniques help release restrictions between cranium and sacrum.

Author details

Siddharth Mehta
Department of Orthodontics, Mahatma Gandhi Dental College and Hospital, MGUMST, Jaipur, India

*Address all correspondence to: sidmehta100@gmail.com

References

[1] Okeson JP. Management of Temporomandibular Disorders and Occlusion. 7 th ed. St. Louis: Elsevier; 2020. ISBN: 978-0-323-58210-0

[2] Kandaswamy S, Rinchuse DJ, Greene CS, Johnston LE Jr. Temporomandibular disorders and orthodontists: What we have learned from 1992-2022? American Journal of Orthodontics and Dentofacial Orthopedics. 7 Jan 2022;**S0889-5406**(21):00831-00833. DOI: 10.1016/j.ajodo.2021.12.011

[3] Ul-Huqh MZ, Hassan R, Azhar MI, Rahman RA, Asif JA, Yusof A, et al. Effect of orthodontic treatment on temporomandibular joint: A review. European Journal of Molecular & Clinical Medicine. 2020;**7**(11):1000-1010

[4] Michelotti A, Rongo R. Orthodontics, and Temporomandibular disorders: Cutting edge of current evidence. Journal of the World Federation of Orthodontists. 2020;**9**:515-518

[5] Yap AU, Zhang MJ, Cao Y, Lei J, Fu KY. Comparison of psychological states and oral health-related quality of life of patients with differing severity of temporomandibular disorders. Journal of Oral Rehabilitation. 2022;**49**(2):177-185

[6] Yap AU, Cao Y, Zhang MJ, Lei J, Fu KY. Comparison of emotional disturbance, sleep, and life quality in adult patients with painful temporomandibular disorders of different origins. Clinical Oral Investigations. 2021;**25**(6):4097-4105

[7] Serritella E, Galluccio G, Impellizzeri A, Di Giacomo P, Di Paolo C. Comparison of the effectiveness of three different acupuncture methods for TMD-related pain: A randomized clinical study. Evidence-based Complementary and Alternative Medicine. 2021;**2021**(30):1286570

[8] Valesan LF, Da-Cas CD, Réus JC, Denardin ACS, Garanhani RR, Bonotto D, et al. Prevalence of temporomandibular joint disorders: A systematic review and meta-analysis. Clinical Oral Investigations. 2021;**25**(2):441-453

[9] Michelotti A, Iodice G. The role of orthodontics in temporomandibular disorders. Journal of Oral Rehabilitation. 2010;**37**(6):411-429

[10] Conti A, Freitas M, Conti P, Henriques J, Janson G. Relationship between signs and symptoms of temporomandibular disorders and orthodontic treatment: a cross-sectional study. The Angle Orthodontist. 2003;**73**(4):411-417

[11] Bales JM, Epstein JB. The role of malocclusion and orthodontics in temporomandibular disorders. Journal of the Canadian Dental Association. 1994;**60**(10):899-905

Chapter 7

Temporomandibular Disorders of Iatrogenic Etiology

Oleg Slesarev

Abstract

Temporomandibular disorder (TMD) is a heterogeneous chronic systemic disease based on genetic, immunological, anatomical, morphological, and functional disorders of the articulatory norm. The task of the diagnostic stage is to identify direct (inherent in only one nosological form) and indirect (occurring in two or more nosological forms) etiological risks that transform into pathogenetic factors and TMDs. The transformation of the pathogenetic horizon of TMDs does characterize by the implementation of a scenario leading to the formation of three nosological forms of the disease: articular and nonarticular lesions of TMJ, and TMDs of iatrogenic etiology. TMDs of iatrogenic etiology constitute the most severe group of patients. Failure to identify biological, technological, and communication iatrogenic risks at the diagnostic stage is the main reason for triggering TMDs of iatrogenic etiology. The transformation of iatrogenic risks into iatrogenic pathogenetic factors leads to the formation of iatrogenic disease. A specialist working with this group of patients must have the necessary competence to make clinical decisions in the diagnosis, treatment, and rehabilitation of patients of this profile, including maxillofacial surgery and psychological counseling. Timely diagnosis of iatrogenic risks is the only preventive measure that prevents the development of iatrogenic TMDs. The therapy of TMDs of iatrogenic etiology does base on an interdisciplinary approach's principles.

Keywords: temporomandibular disorders, iatrogenic TMDs, pathogenesis of TMDs, diagnosis of TMDs

1. Introduction

Temporomandibular disorders (TMDs) are a group of common non-odontogenic maxillofacial pain syndromes. TMDs are the second most common musculoskeletal disorder resulting in pain, dysfunction, and disability [1]. Epidemiological studies have identified problems associated with TMDs in 25% of the population [2, 3], but only 3–7% of patients seek help [4, 5]. In 70% of cases, the reasons for patients visiting the dentist do associate with pain, impaired movements of the lower jaw, and anatomical and functional changes in the temporomandibular joint [6, 7], which is 3.9% of annual visits from the total number of patients with different profiles [8]. Women, in relation to men, present complaints ranging from 2:1 to 8:1 [9–13]. The multifaceted specific picture of the manifestation of the disease leads to incorrect routing of patients, errors in diagnosis and treatment, and chronicity of the TMJ [3, 14–16].

The frequency of severe disorders accompanied by headache and facial pain and characterized by the urgent need for treatment is 1–2% in children, about 5% in adolescents, and 5–12% in adults [17, 18].

Fifty-eight percent of those who consulted a doctor had a history of 3–5 years, and 16% of them reported no positive response to conservative treatment, resulting in 30–40% of acute cases becoming chronic [19]. The average duration of TMJ was 4.19 years and 5.25 ± 2.91 years, respectively, which characterizes TMJ as a heterogeneous chronic systemic disease. The reasons for the duration of the disease indicate either the lack of treatment due to an undetermined diagnosis or unsuccessful observation by a neurologist for trigeminal neuritis or by an otorhinolaryngologist for otitis media [20–23]. In addition, the disease's symptoms may do associate with centrally mediated and neuroplastic changes in the brain, including dysfunction of the endogenous μ-opioid receptor, one of the central analgesic systems involved in pain perception and analgesia [24].

The prevalence of the analyzed disorders, multifactorial pathogenesis, and therapeutic difficulties in the treatment of TMJ prompted Wieckiewicz et al. [25] to make an effort to describe and systematize current TMJ therapeutic concepts based on DC/TMJ data [26]. Treatment of TMJ is complex and requires special knowledge and skills, and to justify the treatment protocol, it is necessary to formulate a diagnosis that takes into account an interdisciplinary approach [27–29], but most patients seeking help due to TMJ symptoms assess that the treatment has episodic success [23, 30]. A meta-analysis showed that 16% of adults require treatment for TMJ [31]. Moreover, those in need of treatment can divided into those who are indicated for active therapy to eliminate severe symptoms and those who require passive supervision. Manfredini et al. [32] conclude that the specialist treating TMDs must, first of all, be able to differentiate between these two groups of patients. For patients requiring treatment for the symptoms of TMDs, it has been found that noninvasive methods should be preferred. However, the complex structure of TMJ, along with the debilitating nature of the disease at an advanced stage, poses challenges for the development and application of more invasive methods of resolution [19, 33–35].

Murphy [3] analyzed the currently used non-invasive, minimally invasive and fully invasive methods of TMJ treatment, where TMJ disorders are the leading symptom [36]. The ultimate goals of the presented modalities are

- increasing the range of motion of the mandible,
- reducing pain and inflammation in the joints and chewing muscles,
- preventing further degenerative changes in the articular tissues, including direct or indirect damage to the joints.

The successful management of temporomandibular disorders depends on identifying and controlling the contributing factors, including occlusal abnormalities, orthodontic treatment, bruxism and orthopedic instability, macrotrauma and microtrauma, factors like poor health and nutrition, joint laxity, and exogenous estrogen [17, 28].

Global review of research findings by Harper et al. [37] revealed a focus of the flow of clinical diagnostic data in line with the substantiation of two interrelated areas of TMJ therapy: (1) minimization of pain in the maxillofacial region, which is generated and maintained by sensitization mechanisms in the central nervous system; and (2) the need for personalized medicine in providing care to this category of patients.

However, the approach to treating TMDs as a purely dental problem may fail, as a significant proportion of symptoms reflect medical conditions [25, 38], including iatrogenic TMDs [8, 39–41]. Sharma et al. [17] identified factors that increase the risk of temporomandibular disorders are called "Predisposing factors" and those causing the onset of temporomandibular disorders are called "Initiating factors" and factors that interfere with healing or enhance the progression of the temporomandibular disorder are called "Perpetuating factors." Iatrogenic injuries can act as both initiating and predisposing factors. This can occur during any dental procedure in which there is early opening like orthodontic treatment, single-sitting root canal treatment, or relapse, which causes a functional imbalance between the temporomandibular joints, muscles, and occlusion. To avoid this damage to the temporomandibular joint, we should always examine the joint [17]. Determining the features of the pathogenesis of TMDs of iatrogenic etiology is a demanded necessity to treat these disorders and for expert evaluation in the event of doctor–patient conflicts. The formation of iatrogenic TMDs proceeds in several stages. The characterization of iatrogenic TMDs as a multistep process made it possible to identify iatrogenic risks triggering the process of iatrogenesis. Timely identification of iatrogenic risks will prevent the development of the disease along the iatrogenic pathway. Disclosure of the stages of iatrogenesis will make it possible to form the principles of diagnosis and treatment of TMDs within the DC/TMD methodology [42–44].

2. Material and research methods

2.1 Study design

A prospective study of 61 clinical cases of TMD with chronic pain (47 women and 14 men) was carried out. We have identified signs of TMJ recurrence in 92% of clinical cases. Of these, 75% complained of TMJ dysfunction and symptoms of chronic pain syndrome, and 25% of TMJ dysfunction. Against the background of the pain syndrome, phenomenological dysfunctions masked by complaints of other problems were revealed. Patients were observed for 2 years (5 points of observation): at the time of treatment; in 6 months; 1 year; 1 year and 6 months; and 2 years.

2.2 Clinical diagnostics

2.2.1 Scales and indices for assessing temporomandibular disorders

Clinical manifestations of TMDs were analyzed using the instruments of axis II DC/TMJ [45] according to the recommendations of Ohrbach et al. [46]. Axis II includes the evaluation of indicators on several scales:

- Scale SCL-90-R [47] modified by Dworkin and Le Resche [48] assess the presence of specific psychological phenomena characteristic of the psychosomatic structure of the personality.
- The GCPS scale (Graded Chronic Pain Scale) [49] integratively assesses the intensity of chronic pain CPI (Characteristic of Pain Intensity) and the degree of disability due to pain syndrome (five degrees of severity, calculated based on the impact of CPI on: daily activities at home, social activities, and labor activity).
- Temporomandibular index was determined by Pehling et al. [50].

2.2.2 Clinical diagnostics of factors of psychological predisposition of TMJ

The method of interviewing, within the framework of a descriptive approach, carried out clinical diagnostics of psychological phenomena, the type of patient's attitude to the disease and communicative deviations according to Rogers [51].

2.2.3 Clinical diagnosis of myofascial and tendon-muscular trigger points

Identification and qualitative characteristics of trigger points in the muscles and tendon-muscle attachments: m. temporalis; m. masseter; m. pterygoideus lat.; m. geniohyoideus; m. sternocleidomastoideus were carried out according to the criteria established by Simons and Travell [52]. Two indicators were considered: the severity of the local convulsive response (biological response) and the reproducibility of pain in response to palpation of the muscle mass and/or tendon-muscle attachment. The response of the trigger point to the action of the stimulus was assessed in points according to Klineberg and Jagger [53].

Visualization of TMJ elements
Cone beam computed tomography and magnetic resonance imaging
Analysis of received images
Craniometry of tomograms of the temporomandibular joint using an individual anatomical landmark of TMJ structures [54]

Statistical processing of the obtained data was performed using the IBM SPSS 21 package and included comparisons of related groups by the Friedman analysis and the paired Wilcoxon test; independent groups by the Mann–Whitney–Wilcoxon test, qualitative signs—analysis of contingency tables by Pearson's chi-square test.

3. Temporomandibular disorders of iatrogenic etiology

- According to our study, 30% of patients presenting with TMJ problems have iatrogenic TMDs. We suppose that a large proportion of patients with iatrogenic TMDs come to our maxillofacial surgery clinic and dentistry because patients with complicated forms of TMDs refer to us. Complications are formed as a result of diagnostic errors, which leads to incorrect formulation of the final diagnosis and incorrect treatment planning.

3.1 Theoretical foundations of the system-structural analysis of the etiology and pathogenesis of temporomandibular disorders

Temporomandibular disorders are heterogeneous chronic systemic diseases based on the articulatory norm's genetic, immunological, anatomical, morphological, and functional disorders. TMD is a symptom complex, the heterogeneity of which is characterized by a fluctuation of clinical symptoms, with periodic dominance of one of them. The pathogenesis of TMDs ends with the formation of specific pathological disorders in the articulation system:

- functional disintegration of the combined functions of the elements of the articulation system and violation of the criteria of the articulation norm;

- pathological occlusion of the dentition in the stage of decompensation;

- combined anatomical and morphological changes in the bone, cartilage, and tendon-muscular structures of the TMJ.

The articulation system is formed by bones of the facial part of the skull, TMJ, chewing muscles, hyoid bone, and dentition in one of the types of physiological occlusion. The anatomical and functional criteria that provide the articulation system's physiological, cosmetic, and phonetic capabilities do realize within the articulation norm's phonetically determined boundaries. Therefore, anatomical and functional criteria of the articulatory norm do determine phylogenesis.

Identifying iatrogenic etiological risks (IERs) that form violations of anatomical and functional relationships in the articulation system is the main task of diagnosing TMDs. Iatrogenic etiological risks are preclinical forms of TMDs (predictors). However, undiagnosed preclinical forms transform into iatrogenic pathogenic factors and, further, into clinical forms of TMDs of iatrogenic etiology. As a result of the transformation, a new set of pathomorphological relationships do form, which clinically manifests itself as a newly formed symptom complex—TMDs (**Table 1**).

Temporomandibular disorders		
Congenital		**Acquired**
Soft tissue pathology: 1. Connective tissue dysplasia syndrome. 2. Polymorphism of the SLC6A4 gene (control of the transmission of nerve impulses using serotonin)	1. Pathology of the development of the bones of the facial part of the skull. 2. Violation of the anatomical ratios of the bones of the facial part of the skull.	1. Pain syndrome: A. Idiopathic pain disorders (violation of nociceptive sensation control systems); B. Functional (violation of the efficiency of signal transmission in the synapse) and morphological (decrease in the volume of gray matter) neuroplastic changes in various parts of the CNS. 2. The impossibility of transferring the lower jaw to the posterior contact position for diagnostic and therapeutic purposes. 3. Violation of the four conditions of functional occlusion [55]. 4. Iatrogenic: A. Inadequate planning of the volume of treatment (an attempt to use conservative methods when indicating a solution to the problem with surgical techniques); B. Functional and anatomical disorders in the TMJ in violation of the bite stability in the lateral sections of the dentition; C. Violation of indications and principles of construction and reorganization of methods of occlusive therapy; D. Violation of the vector of muscle forces that determine the movements of the lower jaw, the nonphysiological ratio of the lower and upper jaws.

Table 1.
The structure of clinically detected etiological factors in the pathogenesis of temporomandibular disorders.

3.2 Etiology and pathogenesis of iatrogenic TMDs

TMDs of iatrogenic etiology have a multicomponent pathogenetic structure. To determine the set of heterogeneous data in the clinical picture of TMDs, we used a system-structural analysis. This will make it possible to identify the paths of pathogenetic transformation of preclinical forms of TMDs into iatrogenic disease (**Figure 1**). Preclinical forms are predictors of TMDs of iatrogenic etiology, which we have classified as iatrogenic etiological risks.

Unidentified iatrogenic etiological risks (IERs) remain at the risk level until the treatment phase. Implementing incorrectly planned therapy brings the IER out of the "sleep state." The transition of preclinical forms of TMDs from the level of IER to the level of iatrogenic pathogenetic factors (IPFs) begins. IPF trigger the iatrogenic disease. Thus, TMDs of iatrogenic etiology result from the transformation of iatrogenic etiological risks into iatrogenic pathogenic factors and iatrogenic disease (**Table 2**).

Failure to identify iatrogenic etiological risks at the diagnostic stage leads to incorrect therapy planning for TMDs. IER predictors are biological, technological, and communicational (psychosocial) forms of risk (**Figure 1**). IERs do not run in isolation and mutually overlap each other.

Biological risks account for 85% of the total share of risks. They are formed in ontogeny and should do identified at the diagnostic stage. According to the level of violations, we single out iatrogenic biological risks of the macrosystem and intrasystem levels.

Biological iatrogenic risks at the macrosystem level:

1. violations of the constants of the anatomical and functional ratio of the bones of the facial and cerebral skulls determined in phylogenesis;

2. the resulting vector of movements of the lower jaw in three cephalometric planes, which ensures the stability of the position of the center of rotation of the lower jaw (f. mandibulae) in space;

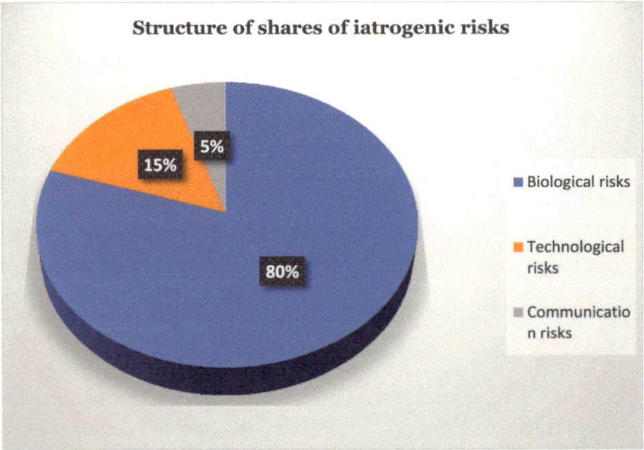

Figure 1.
Structure of shares of iatrogenic risks.

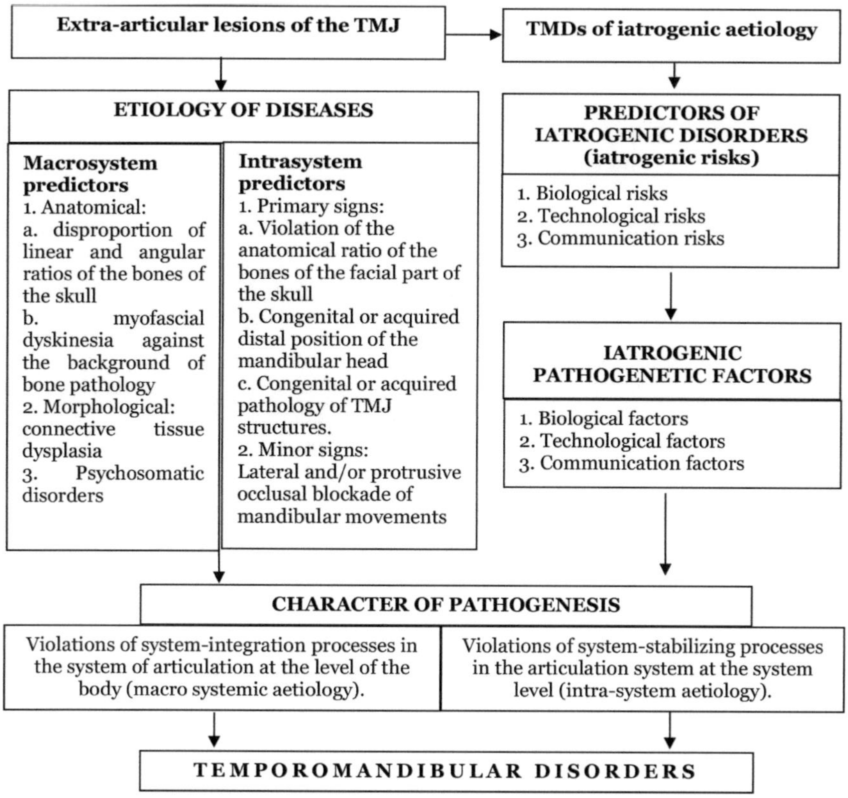

Table 2.
Pathways of pathogenetic transformation of nosological forms—Precursors of TMDs.

3. phenotypic manifestations of clinical markers of undifferentiated forms of connective tissue dysplasia at the macrosystem level (asthenic body type; deformation of the musculoskeletal system; arachnodactyly; degree of skin extensibility; longitudinal and transverse flat feet; refractive error; and nephroptosis);

4. psychological factors involved in the formation of the structure of the disorder's pathogenesis.

Biological iatrogenic risks of intrasystem level:

1. anatomical – metric inconsistencies in the size and shape of the jaws; asymmetry in the size of the branch and body of the lower jaw; and the distal position of the mandibular heads.

2. functional – myofascial dyskinesia of masticatory muscles and active and latent trigger points in the masticatory muscles.

3. occlusal – violation of static and dynamic contacts of the dentition of various origins, and violation of the clinical stages of occlusion equilibration.

4. signs of undifferentiated forms of connective tissue dysplasia at the level of the articulation system: dysfunction of the TMJ; the high vault of the palate; dental anomalies; and short frenulum of the tongue.

Technological iatrogenic risks result from a violation of the protocol for examining a patient with TMDs at the diagnostic stage. For example, insufficient volume examination does not correctly collect the necessary diagnostic data, based on which the final diagnosis does formulate and treatment does plan. In such cases, the decision on the method of treating the disease and, in particular, the use of medical technologies to correct the contact of the dentition, the ratio of the jaws, and the function of the masticatory muscles is methodologically incorrect. Therefore, it leads to the development of iatrogenic disease.

Phenomenological dysfunctions constitute a significant component of communication iatrogenic risks. Communication iatrogenic risks are formed at the stage of diagnosis and manifest themselves in the form of a high level of treatment success expected by the patient, formed by the doctor. Unjustified expectations built into previous consultations form a communication gap between doctor and patient. TMD is a multifactorial disease based on reliably identified risk factors – phenomenological dysfunctions, complicated by psychosomatic disorders that prevail over peripheral nociceptive factors.

When formulating a diagnosis and choosing a medical technology, all unknown iatrogenic etiological risks transform into iatrogenic pathogenetic factors and, in association with other already identified clinical symptoms, form a new symptom complex – TMDs of iatrogenic etiology. Thus, at a new stage in the development of the disease, pathogenetic iatrogenic factors formed from iatrogenic pathogenetic risks are revealed. In the structure of the pathogenesis of iatrogenic TMDs, there is a change in the share of influence of pathogenetic iatrogenic factors – biological factors give way to technological factors (**Figure 2**). This is the result of the hidden influence of unknown iatrogenic risks on the pathogenesis of the disease and the implemented therapeutic and technological solutions. The implemented medical technology aggravates the disease and forms new TMDs of iatrogenic etiology.

4. Conclusions

Thus, in order to avoid such complications as TMDs of iatrogenic etiology in one's practice, it is necessary at the diagnostic stage to identify preclinical forms of TMDs that can initiate the development of iatrogenic disease. Incorrect use of diagnostic methods and procedures is the leading cause of the occurrence and development of iatrogenic TMDs.

Biological risks not identified at the diagnostic stage at the treatment planning stage become the cause of iatrogenic pathogenetic factors and iatrogenic disease. If iatrogenic etiological risks are not identified and do not define as symptoms, they do not consider when formulating a diagnosis or choosing a medical technology. The diagnostic stage is the stage of missed opportunities, at which it is possible to avoid the occurrence of iatrogenic disease. Therefore, the diagnostic stage tests the professional competencies of the clinic. Thus, undiagnosed iatrogenic risks cause the formation of iatrogenic pathogenic factors, the failure to identify which leads to an incorrectly formulated or preliminary clinical diagnosis, treatment plan, negative outcome of therapy, and iatrogenic TMDs. Incorrect diagnosis > incorrect diagnosis > incorrect

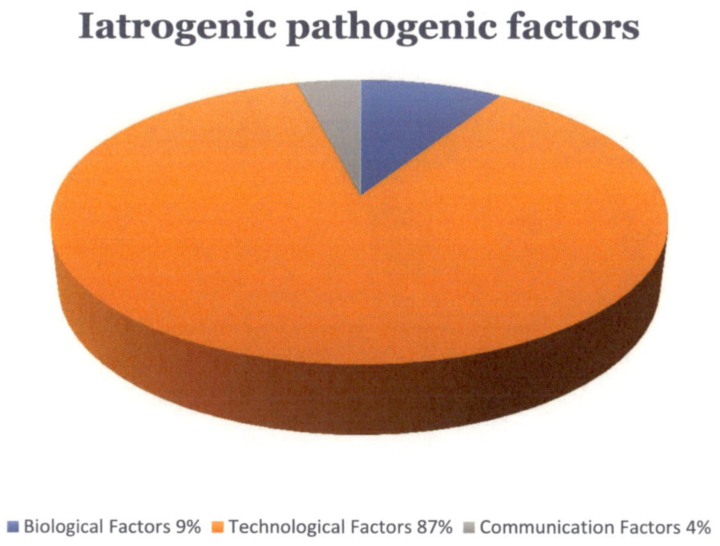

Figure 2.
Structure of shares of iatrogenic pathogenic factors.

choice of medical technology > TMDs of iatrogenic etiology. Timely diagnosis of iatrogenic risks is the main preventive measure that prevents the development of iatrogenic TMDs.

5. Clinical example

Patient K does treat in a previous clinic with a diagnosis of TMDs. She received occlusal therapy using a disengaging occlusal splint (**Figure 3**).

She does admit to our clinic with complaints of limited mouth opening, facial pain, and tooth contact problems. Using DC/TMD tools, we conducted a comprehensive examination of the functional and anatomical state of the articulation system and the psychosocial sphere. Examination of the CBCT of the TMJ with and without an occlusal splint revealed distal position and deformity of the TMJ head surfaces. MRI of the TMJ revealed an unreduced disk dislocation with ligament rupture (**Figures 4** and **5**).

Using an occlusal uncoupling splint in the mandible resulted in destabilization of the TMJ heads, displacement of the TMJ disk into an anterior-internal position, and a sizeable horizontal-to-vertical dentition ratio. Thus, the insufficient amount of applied methods for visualizing TMJ structures without considering data on soft tissue elements obtained by MRI is the cause of a diagnostic error, an incorrect diagnosis, and unreasonable treatment planning. Occlusal therapy uses an occlusal splint, which does indicate in preparation for the surgical solution of the problem, and not as the leading therapeutic solution (**Figure 3**).

Final clinical diagnosis: Deforming arthrosis of the TMJ; unreduced anterior dislocation of the TMJ disk on the right and subluxation on the left; the distal position of the heads of the lower jaw; instability of occlusion in the area of 4.4, 4.5, and 4.6 teeth with a decrease in bite height. Moderate anxiety. First-degree disability.

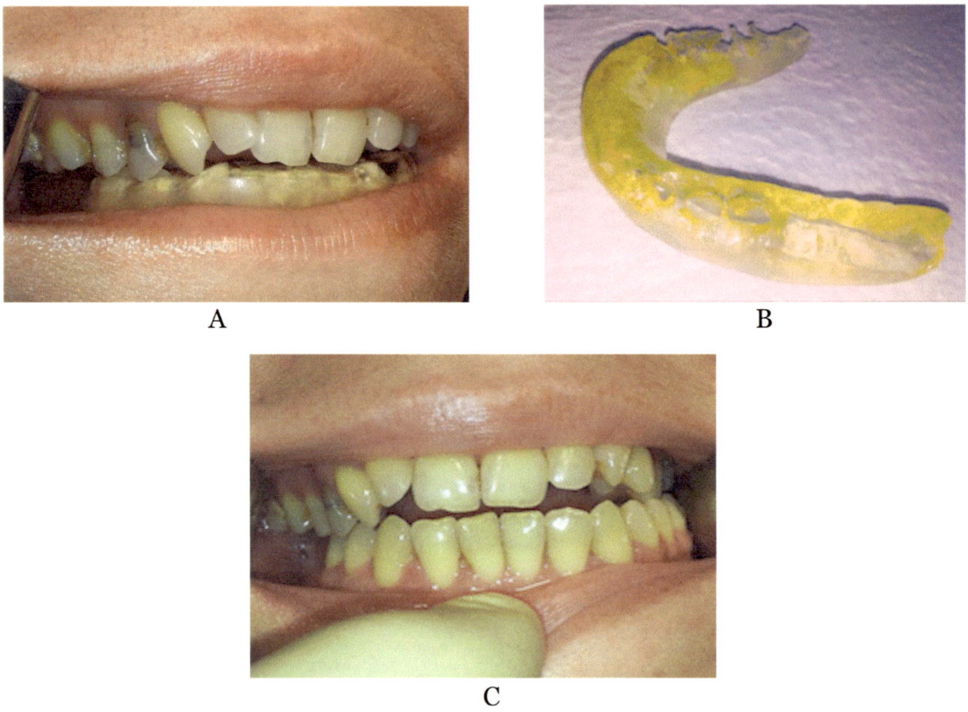

Figure 3.
Photo of patient K. Phantom bite formed by an occlusal splint. A – An occlusal disconnecting tire is superimposed on the lower dentition; B – Occlusal slave splint removed from the oral cavity; C – The position of the dentition in the intertubercular position, a phantom bite is formed.

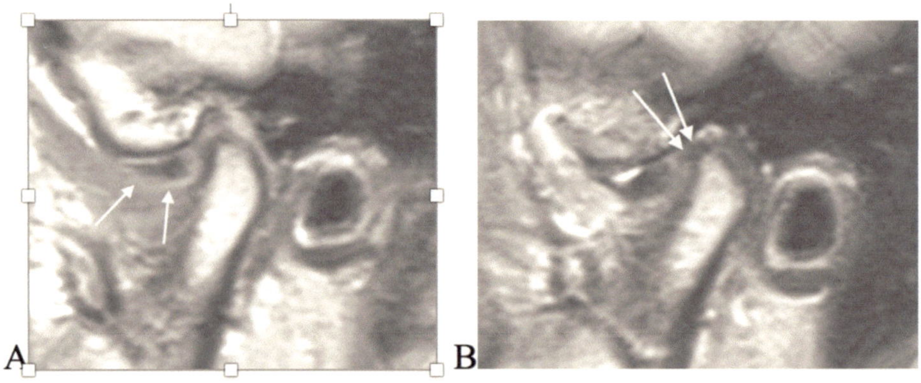

Figure 4.
MRI of the TMJ. A – Anterolateral location of the disk without reduction (↑ ↑ ↑) in the left TMJ. B – Anterolateral disk location without reduction with partial rupture of the posterior discotemporal ligament (↑ ↑ ↑) of the right TMJ.

An unreasonable attempt to eliminate anatomical and functional disorders of the jaw ratio by separating the dentition led to the transformation of the IER in the direction of the IPF. For this reason, the phantom bite of iatrogenic etiology and TMDs of iatrogenic etiology have formed. We identified primary etiological factors (iatrogenic biological risks and anatomical pathogenetic factors, i.e. mismatch of the

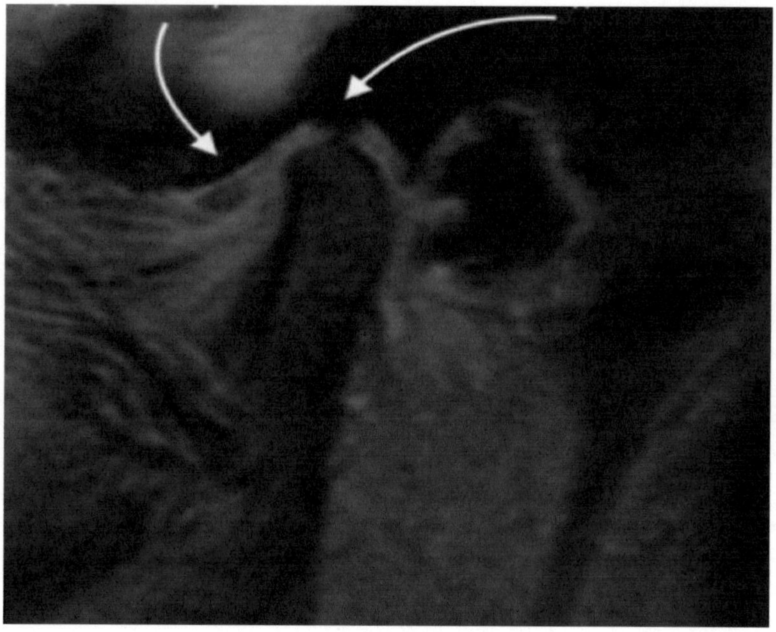

Figure 5.
MRI of the TMJ. Rupture of the posterior ligaments of the TMJ disk.

anatomical size, shape, and position of the bones of the facial part of the skull) and secondary etiological factors (crowded position and disruption of dynamic and static contacts of the teeth). The use of an occlusal disconnecting splint led to disk rupture and forced bite formation. In such clinical cases, it is impossible to compensate for anatomical (organ) risks by affecting only occlusal risks, changing the interocclusal height without considering the horizontal-vertical ratio of the dentition. Therefore, it does decide to prepare for reorganizing occlusal therapy with an occlusal stabilizing splint, provisional prosthetics, and pharmacotherapy in combination with CBPC. The use of an occlusal stabilizing splint makes it possible to stabilize the horizontal-vertical ratio of the jaws to model and carry out intraoral verification of occlusal guiding movements of the lower jaw in the protrusion and laterotrusion directions.

Failure to identify iatrogenic biological risks of the macrosystem and intrasystem levels in the patient led to an incorrect diagnosis formulation and incorrect therapy planning. The splint design does make on the lower jaw dentition without considering the vertical-horizontal ratio of the jaws, protrusion, and laterotrusion guides. Overlapping the frontal group of teeth with a splint led to the distalization of the lower jaw. After 2 years of wearing the splint, a phantom bite developed, characterized by lower jaw distalization, occlusion instability, pain syndrome, and TMJ dysfunction.

The use of dissociating occlusal devices, the manufacture of which did not consider the anatomical and functional conditions of occlusal guiding movements of the lower jaw in the protrusion and laterotrusion directions in conjunction with the horizontal-vertical ratio of the jaws, is the cause of the formation of two types of iatrogenies:

1. Iatrogenia are formed by a dissociating occlusal splint and superimposed on the lower jaw with overlapping of the occlusal surface of the teeth of the frontal section. The frontal occlusal platform, when the dentition is closed, slides along

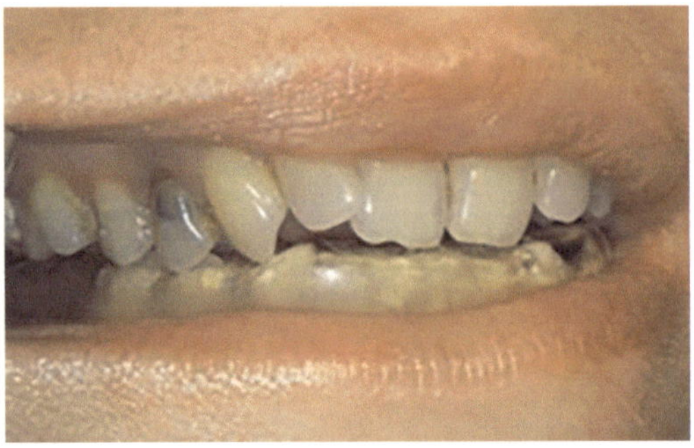

Figure 6.
Photo of the dentition of the patient P. Disconnecting occlusal tire on the lower dentition with overlapping of the frontal group of teeth.

the palatal surface of the incisors of the upper jaw and moves the lower jaw distally to a distance corresponding to the amount of desocclusion, i.e. the thickness of the overlap of the lower jaw incisors by the occlusal platform, which leads to a change in the excursions of the TMJ heads and the transfer of the load vector from vector to tangential. This causes pathological mobility, and frontal dislocation of the upper anterior group of teeth causes gum recession in the lower jaw (**Figure 6**).

When visualizing the TMJ by CT, the distal position of the heads is revealed with a critical approach to the neurovascular bundle in the petrotympanic fissure. The nature of the movements of the head of the lower jaw changes: it performs only rotational movements, the stage of sliding down and forward is replaced by a horizontal movement toward the slope of the tubercle. When visualizing soft tissue elements by MRI in all functional positions, anterior, at 8 or 10 o'clock, disk displacement is diagnosed, which leads to the formation of disk dislocation without self-reduction. The posterior ligaments of the disk experience pathological stresses, stretch, and lose their ability to regulate disk excursions.

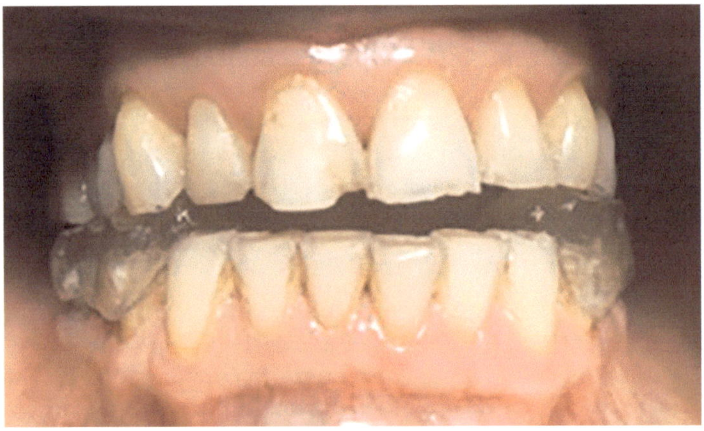

Figure 7.
Photo of patient E's teeth with an occlusal disconnecting splint made on the lower dentition without considering the occlusal guiding movements of the lower jaw in the frontal and laterotrusive planes. View at the initial visit after treatment for 2 years in another clinic.

The vascular-nervous elements in the bilaminar zone experience compression of the TMJ head, which leads to fluid effusion in this area, the formation of a pain syndrome, a decrease in hearing acuity, and a symptom of a foreign body in the middle ear.

2. Iatrogenia are formed as a result of anatomically unreasonable use of an uncoupling occlusal device in the area of the chewing group of teeth. There is a loss of occlusal guides and the posterior contact position of the mandible (**Figure** 7). On CT, this is manifested by the displacement of the head of the mandible vertically downward and backward. MRI shows disk rupture, tear, and overstretching of the TMJ ligaments.

Conflict of interest

The authors declare no conflict of interest.

Author details

Oleg Slesarev
Samara State Medical University, Samara, Russia

*Address all correspondence to: o.slesarev@gmail.com

References

[1] Schiffman EL, Ahmad M, Hollender L, Kartha K, Ohrbach R, Truelove EL, et al. Longitudinal stability of common TMJ structural disorders. Journal of Dental Research. 2017;**96**(3):270-276. DOI: 10.1177/0022034516679396

[2] Manfredini D, Lombardo L, Siciliani GJ. Temporomandibular disorders and dental occlusion. A systematic review of association studies: End of an era? Oral Rehabilitation. 2017;**44**(11):908-923

[3] Murphy MK, MacBarb RF, Wong ME, Athanasiou KA. Temporomandibular disorders: A review of etiology, clinical management, and tissue engineering strategies. The International Journal of Oral & Maxillofacial Implants. 2013;**28** (6):e393-e414. DOI: 10.11607/jomi.te20

[4] Carlsson GE. Epidemiology and treatment need for temporomandibular disorders. Journal of Orofacial Pain. 1999;**13**(4):232-237

[5] Gauer RL, Semidey MJ. Diagnosis and treatment of temporomandibular disorders. American Family Physician. 2015;**91**(6):378-386

[6] Paniagua B, Pascal L, Prieto J, et al. Diagnostic index: An open-source tool to classify TMJ OA condyles. Proceedings of SPIE – The International Society for Optical Engineering. 2017;**10137**: 101372H. DOI: 10.1117/12.2254070

[7] Embree MC, Iwaoka GM, Kong D, Martin BN, Patel RK, Lee AH, et al. Soft tissue ossification and condylar cartilage degeneration following TMJ disc perforation in a rabbit pilot study. Osteoarthritis and Cartilage. 2015;**23**(4): 629-639. DOI: 10.1016/j.joca.2014.12.015

[8] Slade GD, Ohrbach R, Greenspan JD, Fillingim RB, Bair E, Sanders AE, et al. Painful temporomandibular disorder: Decade of discovery from OPPERA studies. Journal of Dental Research. 2016;**95**(10):1084-1092. DOI: 10.1177/0022034516653743

[9] Gonçalves DA, Camparis CM, Speciali JG, Franco AL, Castanharo SM, Bigal ME. Temporomandibular disorders are differentially associated with headache diagnoses: A controlled study. The Clinical Journal of Pain. 2011;**27**(7): 611-615. DOI: 10.1097/AJP.0b013e31820e12f5

[10] Iwasaki LR, Gonzalez YM, Liu Y, Liu H, Markova M, Gallo LM, et al. TMJ energy densities in healthy men and women. Osteoarthritis and Cartilage. 2017;**25**(6):846-849. DOI: 10.1016/j.joca.2016.12.027

[11] Iwasaki LR, Gonzalez YM, Liu Y, et al. Mechanobehavioral scores in women with and without TMJ disc displacement. Journal of Dental Research. 2017;**96**(8):895-901. DOI: 10.1177/0022034517704375

[12] Wright EF, North SL. Management and treatment of temporomandibular disorders: A clinical perspective. The Journal of Manual and Manipulative Therapy. 2009;**17**(4):247-254. DOI: 10.1179/106698109791352184

[13] Ahmad M, Schiffman EL. Temporomandibular joint disorders and orofacial pain. Dental Clinics of North America. 2016;**60**(1):105

[14] Chantaracherd P, John MT, Hodges JS, Schiffman EL. Temporomandibular joint disorders' impact on pain, function, and disability. Journal of Dental Research. 2015;**94**(3 Suppl):79S-86S. DOI: 10.1177/0022034514565793

[15] Ebrahim FH, Ruellas ACO, Paniagua B, et al. Accuracy of biomarkers obtained from cone beam computed tomography in assessing the internal trabecular structure of the mandibular condyle. Oral Surgery, Oral Medicine, Oral Pathology and Oral Radiology. 2017; **124**(6):588-599. DOI: 10.1016/j.oooo.2017.08.013

[16] Poluha RL, Canales GT, Costa YM, Grossmann E, Bonjardim LR, Conti PCR. Temporomandibular joint disc displacement with reduction: A review of mechanisms and clinical presentation. Journal of Applied Oral Science. 2019; **27**:e20180433. DOI: 10.1590/1678-7757-2018-0433 Erratum in: Journal of Applied Oral Science. 2019;27: e2019er001

[17] Sharma S, Gupta DS, Pal US, Jurel SK. Etiological factors of temporomandibular joint disorders. National Journal of Maxillofacial Surgery. 2011;**2**(2):116-119. DOI: 10.4103/0975-5950.94463

[18] Athanasiou AE. Orthodontics and craniomandibular disorders. In: Samire B, editor. Textbook of Orthodontics. 2nd ed. Philadelphia: Saunders; 2003. pp. 478-493

[19] Wolford LM, Mercuri LG, Schneiderman ED, Movahed R, Allen W. Twenty-year follow-up study on a patient-fitted temporomandibular joint prosthesis: The Techmedica/TMJ concepts device. Journal of Oral & Maxillofacial Surgery. 2015;**73**(5): 952-960. DOI: 10.1016/j.joms.2014.10.032

[20] Ceusters W, Michelotti A, Raphael KG, Durham J, Ohrbach R. Perspectives on next steps in classification of oro-facial pain—Part 1: Role of ontology. Journal of Oral Rehabilitation. 2015; **42**(12):926-941. DOI: 10.1111/joor.12336

[21] Shueb SS, Nixdorf DR, John MT, Alonso BF, Durham J. What is the impact of acute and chronic orofacial pain on quality of life? Journal of Dentistry. 2015;**43**(10):1203-1210. DOI: 10.1016/j.jdent.2015.06.001

[22] Okeson JP. Evolution of occlusion and temporomandibular disorder in orthodontics: Past, present, and future. American Journal of Orthodontics & Dentofacial Orthopedics. 2015;**147**(5 Suppl):S216-S223

[23] O'Keeffe M, O'Sullivan PB, O'Sullivan K. Education can 'change the world': Can clinical education change the trajectory of individuals with back pain? British Journal of Sports Medicine. 2019; **53**:1385-1386

[24] van Steenbergen H, Eikemo M, Leknes S. The role of the opioid system in decision making and cognitive control: A review. Cognitive, Affective, & Behavioral Neuroscience. 2019;**19**(3):435-458. DOI: 10.3758/s13415-019-00710-6

[25] Wieckiewicz M, Boening K, Wiland P, Shiau YY, Paradowska-Stolarz A. Reported concepts for the treatment modalities and pain management of temporomandibular disorders. The Journal of Headache & Pain. 2015;**16**: 106. DOI: 10.1186/s10194-015-0586-5

[26] Schiffman E, Ohrbach R, Truelove E, Look J, Anderson G, Goulet JP, et al. Diagnostic criteria for temporomandibular disorders (DC/TMD) for clinical and research applications: Recommendations of the International RDC/TMD Consortium Network and Orofacial Pain Special Interest Group. Journal of Oral & Facial Pain and Headache. 2014;**28**(1):6-27. DOI: 10.11607/jop.1151

[27] Miernik M, Wieckiewicz M, Paradowska A, Wieckiewicz W. Massage

therapy in myofascial TMD pain management. Advances in Clinical Experimental Medicine. 2012;**21**(5): 681-685

[28] Ohrbach R, Dworkin SF. The evolution of TMD diagnosis: Past, present, future. Journal of Dental Research. 2016;**95**(10):1093-1101. DOI: 10.1177/0022034516653922

[29] Dinsdale A, Liang Z, Thomas L, Treleaven J. Are jaw range of motion, muscle function and proprioception impaired in adults with persistent temporomandibular disorders? A systematic review and meta-analysis. Journal of Oral Rehabilitation. 2020; **47**:1448-1478

[30] Wänman A, Marklund S. Treatment outcome of supervised exercise, home exercise and bite splint therapy, respectively, in patients with symptomatic disc displacement with reduction: A randomised clinical trial. Journal of Oral Rehabilitation. 2019; **47**:143-149

[31] Manfredini D, Segù M, Arveda N, et al. Temporomandibular joint disorders in patients with different facial morphology. A systematic review of the literature. Journal of Oral & Maxillofacial Surgery. 2016;**74**:29-46

[32] Tresoldi M, Dias R, Bracci A, Segù M, Guarda-Nardini L, Manfredini D. Magnetic resonance imaging evaluation of closed-mouth TMJ disc-condyle relationship in a population of patients seeking for temporomandibular disorders advice. Pain Research and Management. 2021;**2021**:8. Article ID 5565747. DOI: 10.1155/2021/5565747

[33] Folle FS, Poluha RL, Setogutti ET, Grossmann E. Double puncture versus single puncture arthrocentesis for the management of unilateral temporomandibular joint disc displacement without reduction: A randomized controlled trial. Journal of Cranio-Maxillo-Facial Surgery. 2018; **46**(12):2003-2007. DOI: 10.1016/j.jcms.2018.10.015

[34] Warburton G. Internal derangements of the temporomandibular joint. In: Bonanthaya K, Panneerselvam E, Manuel S, Kumar VV, Rai A, editors. Oral and Maxillofacial Surgery for the Clinician. Singapore: Springer; 2021. DOI: 10.1007/978-981-15-1346-6_63

[35] Vicente González L, Pablo López J, Díaz-Báez D, Gómez-Delgado A. Correlation between MRI-diagnosed joint effusion and demographic, clinical, imaging, and arthroscopic findings of the temporomandibular joint. Journal of Cranio-Maxillofacial Surgery. 2021; **49**(12):1169-1174

[36] Tchivileva IE, Hadgraft H, Lim PF, Di Giosia M, Ribeiro-Dasilva M, Campbell JH, et al. Efficacy and safety of propranolol for treatment of temporomandibular disorder pain: A randomized, placebo-controlled clinical trial. Pain. 2020;**161**(8):1755-1767. DOI: 10.1097/j.pain.0000000000001882

[37] Harper DE, Schrepf A, Clauw DJ. Pain mechanisms and centralized pain in temporomandibular disorders. Journal of Dental Research. 2016;**95**(10):1102-1108. DOI: 10.1177/0022034516657070

[38] Ringold S, Weiss PF, Colbert RA, DeWitt EM, Lee T, Onel K, et al. Childhood arthritis and rheumatology research alliance consensus treatment plans for new-onset polyarticular juvenile idiopathic arthritis. Arthritis Care & Research (Hoboken). 2014;**66**(7):1063-1072. DOI: 10.1002/acr.22259

[39] Alamir AH, Hakami YA, Alabsi FS, et al. Potential myogenous temporomandibular disorders following iatrogenic occlusal disturbance: A pilot study. The Journal of Contemporary Dental Practice. 2019; **20**(10):1138-1140

[40] Slade GD, Akinkugbe AA, Sanders AE. Projections of U.S. edentulism prevalence following 5 decades of decline. Journal of Dental Research. 2014;**93**(10):959-965. DOI: 10.1177/0022034514546165

[41] Furquim BD, Flamengui LM, Conti PC. TMD and chronic pain: A current view. Dental Press Journal of Orthodontics. 2015;**20**(1):127-133. DOI: 10.1590/2176-9451.20.1.127-133.sar

[42] Schiffman E, Ohrbach R, Truelove E, Look J, Anderson G, Goulet JP, et al. Diagnostic criteria for temporomandibular disorders (DC/TMD) for clinical and research applications: Recommendations of the International RDC/TMD Consortium Network and Orofacial Pain Special Interest Group. Journal of Oral & Facial Pain. 2014;**28**(1):6-27. DOI: 10.11607/jop.1151

[43] Rongo R et al. Diagnostic criteria for temporomandibular disorders (DC/TMD) for children and adolescents: An international Delphi study—Part 1—Development of Axis I. Journal of Oral Rehabilitation. 2021;**48**:836-884. DOI: 10.1111/joor.1317

[44] Rongo R, Ekberg E, Nilsson IM, et al. Diagnostic criteria for temporomandibular disorders (DC/TMD) in children and adolescents: An international Delphi study—Part 2—Development of Axis II. Journal of Oral Rehabilitation. 2021;**49**(5):541-552. DOI: 10.1111/joor.13301

[45] Ohrbach R, Turner JA, Sherman JJ, et al. The research diagnostic criteria for temporomandibular disorders. IV: Evaluation of psychometric properties of the Axis II measures. Journal of Orofacial Pain. 2010;**24**(1):48-62

[46] Ohrbach R, List T, Goulet JP, Svensson P. Recommendations from the International Consensus Workshop: Convergence on an Orofacial pain taxonomy. Journal of Oral Rehabilitation. 2010 In press

[47] Derogatis LR, Lipman RS, Covi L. SCL-90: An outpatient psychiatric rating scale—Preliminary report. Psychopharmacology Bulletin. 1973;**9**:13-28

[48] Dworkin SF, Le Resche L. Research diagnostic criteria for temporomandibular disorders: Review, criteria, examinations and specifications, critique. Journal of Craniomandibular Disorders: Facial & Oral Pain. 1992;**6**:301-355

[49] Von Korff M, Ormel J, Keefe FJ, et al. Grading the severity of chronic pain. Pain. 1992;**50**:133-149

[50] Pehling J et al. Interexaminer reliability and clinical validity of the temporomandibular index: A new outcome measure for temporomandibular disorders. Journal of Orofacial Pain. 2002;**16**(4):296-304

[51] Rogers RC. The Art of Counseling and Therapy. M.: Aprel' Press, izd-voJeksmo; 2002 (976 s. In Russ.) English translation O. Kondrashovoj, R. Kuchkarovoj, T. Rozhkovoj, Ju. Ovchinnikovoj, G. Pimochkinoj, M. Zlotnik.

[52] Simons DG, Travell JG, Simons LS, Travell JG. Travell & Simons' Myofascial Pain and Dysfunction: The Trigger Point

Manual. Baltimore: Williams & Wilkins; 1999

[53] Klineberg I, Jagger R, editors. Occlusion and Clinical Practice. M.: MEDPress-inform; 2006 (200 p. il. English translation under general editorship M.M. Antonik, In Russ.)

[54] Slesarev OV. Anatomic rationale and radiological experience in using an individual anatomical landmark during linear imaging of the human temporomandibular joint. Journal of Radiology and Nuclear Medicine. 2014;**3**: 46-51 (In Russ.). DOI: 10.20862/0042-4676-2014-0-3-1-12

[55] Roth RH, Rolfs DA. Functional occlusion for the orthodontist. Part II. Journal of Clinical Orthodontics. 1981; **15**(2):100-123

Chapter 8

Temporomandibular Joint Hypermobility Examination through Differentiation of Sounds

Jolanta E. Loster and Justyna Grochala

Abstract

The temporomandibular joint (TMJ), being an almost well-known anatomical structure but its diagnosis may become difficult due to sounds accompanying joint movement. One example is temporomandibular joint hypermobility (TMJH), which still requires comprehensive study. TMJH is a rare disorder; however, its prevalence at the level of around 4% is still significant. We propose a diagnostic method of TMJH based on the digital time-frequency analysis of sounds generated by TMJ. The volunteers were diagnosed using the RDC/TMD questionnaire and auscultated with the Littmann 3200 electronic stethoscopes on both sides of the head simultaneously. Recorded TMJ sounds were transferred to the computer via Bluetooth® for numerical analysis. The research reveals characteristic time-frequency features in acoustic signals which can be used to detect TMJH. This can help differentiate other disc displacements from joint hypermobility.

Keywords: temporomandibular joint, hypermobility, joint auscultation

1. Introduction

Following the survey carried out in Germany in 2017, the number of cases with temporomandibular joint dislocation as hypermobility movement accounts for 3% of all documented dislocation, which means at least 25 cases per 100,000 inhabitants each year [1]. Following European Commission rules, it could be classified as a rare disease – affecting fewer than 5 people in 10,000 are considered to be so. It is also reported to represent 3% of all dislocated joints cases in the human body. On the other hand, dislocation of temporomandibular joint occurs in up to 7% of people during their lifetime [2]. Shorey and Campbell [3] referred to Sir Astley Cooper's research from the year 1832, who proposed principles for diagnosis and treatment of lower jaw dislocations and introduced nomenclature of joints hypermobility: 'complete dislocation' as luxation and 'imperfect dislocation' as subluxation. The incidences of subluxation are estimated to occur in about 70% of the population based on clinical and radiographic analysis [4]. In new classification proposed by Akinbami [5], three types of dislocation based on clinic-radiological evaluation were presented: type I – the head of condyle directly below the tip of the eminence; type II – the head of condyle in the front of the tip of the eminence; type III – the head of condyle located high up

IntechOpen

in the front of base of the eminence. Two types of dislocation with a possibility to self-reduce the hypermobility can be distinguished - subluxation – with, or luxation – without self-reducing.

From The Glossary of Prosthodontic Terms [6], the definition of temporomandibular joint condylar subluxation is: 'self-reducing incomplete or partial dislocation of the condyle', and of incomplete dislocation is: 'a border position of the disk-condyle complex out of the physiological end of movement position in relation to articular eminence'. Partial dislocation is explained in the glossary [6] as a 'displacement of the articular disk resulting in a seriously impaired disk-condyle complex function'. Condylar dislocation [6] is defined as 'a non-self-reducing displacement of the mandibular condyle usually forward of the articular eminence'.

For the condylar displacement, the definition stands as follow – it is when the condyle stands out of the articular eminence in maximal jaw opening position. However, definitions confuse subluxation, luxation and disk displacement. From the clinical point of view, subluxation occurs when the opening of patient's mandibular ends with disk-condyle complex position forward to the articular eminence, which is self-reducing [3]. It means that the patient can close the mandible without any assistance, only by repositioning the mandibular into the disk-condyle complex. It usually concerns joint on one side. With both sides affected it could be more difficult to close the mouth, but patients can usually manage with that on their own. This concerns especially patients with general joints hypermobility, like the Ehlers-Danlos syndrome [7]. They may be frightened or disoriented when it happens for the first time i.e. during yawning. If there is a problem with self-healing and the patient is looking for medical help it could be named as joint dislocation, complete dislocation or luxation. When the dislocation concerns both joints, it looks very dramatic, because patient is unable to speak, swallow and of course, close the mouth. Such cases require medical help, whereas in recurring cases surgical treatment should be considered. It is compatible with Cooper and other authors who followed him, that suggest calling it habitual or recurrent dislocation in cases with more frequent incidents of dislocation and when it is going progressively wrong [3, 8, 9].

As with the other temporomandibular disorders, joint dislocation is often reported by females, especially in recurrent cases. Tendency to dislocation is associated with the shape of anatomical elements like the condyle, glenoid fossa and articular eminence. The pathogenesis is multifactorial, however, for almost 60% of cases, a preceding trauma has been indicated. The mechanism of dislocation also contributes: age, dentition and neurological or neuromuscular diseases. The older the patient, the more he/she is exposed. Lack of posterior teeth support, correlated with advanced tooth loss or edentulous arches without the denture is regarded as favorable to develop joint dislocation. As a recurrent problem for older people with multimorbidity, it significantly reduces their quality of life.

2. Anatomy and physiology

The 'displacement of the articular disk' which is 'non-self-reducing' is usually understood as a pathological position of the disk in relation to the condyle. That pathology is explained as a forward movement of the disk in relation to the condyle (non-reducing), which results in limitations of condylar head movements, and it is often called 'disk lock' or 'disk displacement without reduction'. The main symptoms of that pathology are sudden disappearance of joints sounds, limitation in jaw opening, and lateral jaw displacement during movement, and usually acute pain from the joint region. The above symptoms are opposite to suspected joint subluxation.

From the anatomy of the temporomandibular joints' point of view, it is well known that these joints are extremely complex synovial articulations. In the distal part of the joints — which is in the backside of the disk — exists a bilaminar zone, named also retro-articular structure or hydrodynamic retral pad or retrodiscal tissue [10, 11]. It is a mass of loose, highly vascularized and innervated, connective tissue attached to the posterior edge of the articular disk which extends and fills the loose folds of the posterior capsule of the temporomandibular joint [6]. It changes its position simultaneously with all the disk moves and protects the joints against posteriorly oriented trauma [12]. Although the research of Schmolke [13] carried out on human cadavers has concluded, that it was not possible to distinguish the distal disk as a part of a separated structure, Merida-Velasco et al. [10] reported that after examination of 20 cadavers they have identified two separated laminae and retroarticular region filled with venous plexus. The authors confirmed the presence of discomalleolar ligaments in that region and agreed with suggestion about limitation of the range of opening function by those ligaments [14]. Apparently, that part of the joint capsule is still not fully explored.

During the jaw function, both left and right joints move and they are in mutual interdependence. Going again to the anatomy, joints are divided by the disk into two compartments — the upper and the lower. In that two compartments, different movements take place. The movement in the upper one is mostly translational. In the lower compartment movements are mostly rotational. One of the joint's functions is to connect the mandibular condyle movements in relation to the articular fossa of the temporal bone with the temporomandibular disk interposed. The disk itself is connected with the joint capsule. The capsule is constructed from fibrous ligaments that enclose the joint and limit its motion [15]. It is lined with the synovial membrane.

In order for the movement to be smooth and free of any sound, each surface of the joints, the disks and condylar heads as well as the articular fossae should be sleek and moistened. The articular surfaces are covered by synovial membrane and moistened by synovial fluid. That fluid is produced by specialized endothelial cells capable of producing synovial fluid. It fills all joints' cavities surrounded by the membrane. For proper joints movements, the capsules need to be flexible enough and tight to keep joints parts together during all joints positions [11].

The joints' shifting results in opening, closing, forward, backward and lateral movements of the mandible. During the first four movements, both joints work simultaneously, in mirror reflection. Yet, in the lateral movements, the movement made by the side joint is smaller than the one made by the opposite joint. When one moves, it always results in the movement of the other. That relationship — where one bone (the mandible) moves between two joints, which are mutually dependent on each other — is specific in human skeleton and occurs only in that very specific joints.

Movements are related to joints disks position, capsules and ligaments tension and muscle function. Muscles that are involved in the temporomandibular joint functions are mainly the temporal, masseter, digastricus, medial and lateral pterygoid. From contemporary anatomy, we know that some fibers of temporal, masseter and upper head of lateral pterygoid muscle penetrate to the joint capsule and even to the joint disk [11, 16]. This can result in disk movements, but in the case of muscle hyperactivity could cause disk displacement.

The physiological joints opening movement starts with condyles located in the higher position in relation to the glenoid fossa with the disk between them in the uppermost position. Then, the condyle's head makes a rotation movement in relation to the disk in the lower joint compartment, and the disk translates down and forward in relation to the glenoid fossa and the articular eminence, as a movement in the upper jaw compartment. At the end of the movement, the condyle head is covered by the disk and located on the top of the articular eminence in its lowest possible position. This movement is limited by the joint capsule tension and the ligaments. The bilaminar zone tissues are maximally stretched. In the physiological movement of the joints, the relation between the condyles and the eminences is expected to be the same during the entire action of the opening and closing of the lower jaw. That condyle head position in relation to the fossa and the eminence can be visualized by pantomographic x-ray examination [17].

3. Temporomandibular joint examination opportunities

The diagnostic methods of temporomandibular joint hypermobility are various and there is a possibility to use non-invasive methods such as clinical examination, auscultation, ultrasonography (USG) or magnetic resonance imaging (MRI). It can be also diagnosed by some invasive methods such as X-ray or computed tomography (CT). Clinical examination, X-rays and auscultation are more convenient for the patients and they give enough medical data for proper diagnoses, so there is no need to buy advanced equipment.

Firstly, the clinical examination should be carried out in a repetitive way at every patient [18]. To realize the assumptions a way of examination was thoroughly described in the validated international protocol Diagnostic Criteria for Temporomandibular Disorders (DC/TMD) [19]. It helps to make the examination in a repeatable way and find a proper diagnosis. The stethoscopes are the main instruments for joint auscultation, their advantage is their vast accessibility [20, 21]. The researchers used various modifications of stethoscopes for joints auscultation [22]. The use of a stethoscope, especially an electronic one for examination allows sending the signal via Bluetooth to the computer for further analysis. That tool was used in the research by Wiedmann et al. [23]. Such a method could also help an inexperienced dentist to consult the cases with a specialist. USG of joints region, especially made by an experienced person allows detecting the position of the disk-condyle complex in a dynamic, real way during the test [24]. It informs about the muscle tension, shape of joints compartments and the amount of synovial fluid. This method is non-invasive, repetitive and gives a satisfying amount of information. MRI, belonging also to the non-invasive examination methods, requires dedicated tools and an experienced person for proper interpretation of the results. It can help to detect disc position, the amount of joint fluid and present the bones structures, yet this technique is the most expensive of the non-invasive methods [25].

Computed tomography (CT) belongs to the invasive examination methods and the radiation dose is the biggest. The advantage of this examination is the very precise detection of the properties of the osseous components of the temporomandibular joints [26]. A much lower radiation dose and sufficient amount of clinical data are obtained from an x-ray examination from pantomographs. Currently, they are the very basic equipment of almost all dental offices so diagnostic technic seems to be very easy and common. As the result of that examination, we receive four pictures, two of each side of the face. Two of them present the mandible in the state of closing and the other two in the maximal opening position. The analysis of both sides is possible and easy. Not too many anatomical structures disturb the image. The example of that x-ray is presented in **Figure 1**.

That examination informs us about condyle bone structure, shape and relation to the fossae in maximal intercuspal position and at the end of opening movement. The result of such an x-ray should be compared with patient's clinical status. It is important to analyze the opening and closing jaw movements in relation to upper and lower incisor midline positions during all the movements. The range of openings should be measured between the incisal edges. Then palpation in temporomandibular joints region during mandibular movements and auscultation of that region would be crucial [27].

3.1 Symptoms and diagnosis

Signs and symptoms of acute or chronic dislocation as hypermobility are the same and include temporary inability to close the mouth, preauricular depression of the skin, excessive salivation, tense, spastic muscle of mastication and pain of temporomandibular joint. At the time of a wide opening, specific sounds may appear. It would happen during excessive mouth opening such as yawning, eating, singing or vomiting. The people who are most vulnerable are the ones who suffer from generalized joint hypermobility as Ehlers-Danlos syndrome or Marfan syndrome as well as neurodegenerative/neurodysfunctional diseases or muscle dystrophies [28, 29]. In the described groups of patients, that symptom could be physiological and often that joint hypermobility is painless. Very characteristic in that cases of hypermobility movement are self-reducing, but sometimes the patients are afraid about complications. The problem could also appear after intubation in general anesthesia too. Repeated episodes of subluxation may result in the lengthening of the capsule ligaments or

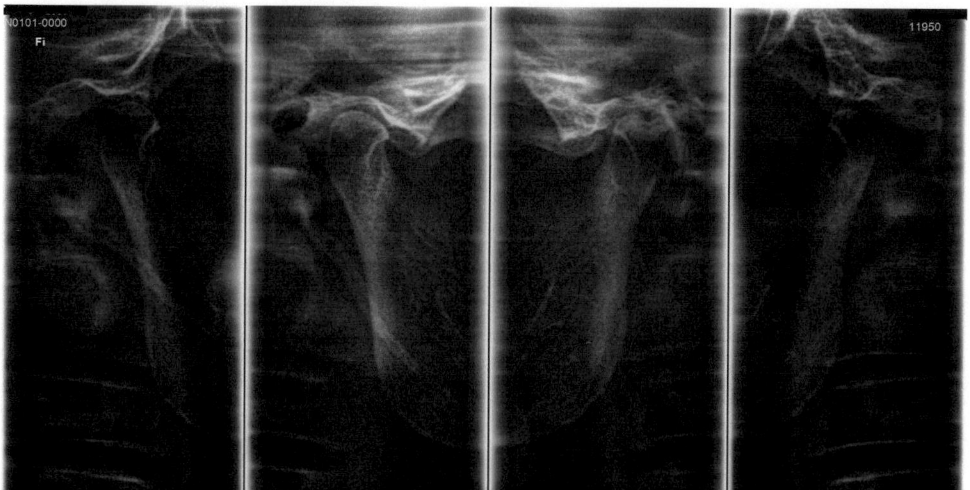

Figure 1.
Right (two left pictures) and left temporomandibular joints in opening (outer images) and closing position with physiological relation of joints elements.

cause damage to the joint capsule. To make the proper diagnosis clinical examination with joint auscultation and x-ray examination are required.

The clinical examination includes the measurement of jaw abduction, lateral movements and protrusion. The symmetry of movements and their straight direction inform us about their proper function. Then the palpation of jaw movement muscle is required. During the examination, muscles should be in the relaxed position. Before palpation, the stretch of the muscle should be investigated. We are expecting symmetrical contraction in the muscles on both sides during the opening and closing of the mandible. Similarly during forward and backward movement. At that moment the tendons and muscle bodies are palpated, especially temporalis, masseter and digastricus. Those muscles are suitable for direct palpation. Lateral pterygoid muscle can be examined using indirect movements. In such a case the examiner's hands should block patient's forward and lateral jaw movements and the doctor should ask the patients about the pain in the region of the joints. The appearance of pain informs about muscle dysfunction, hyperfunction or overactivity [30].

During physiological jaw movements, neither sound nor noises from joints region are expected. If they appear, some disturbances occur i.e. in relation between disk and condylar head or between disk-condyle complex and fossa to articular eminence. The joint dysfunction might be differentiated by sound and it requires auscultating them. Typical sound associated with joints dislocation correlated with hypermobile movement appears at the end of the movement, usually when the mouth is being opened. Subluxation sounds are very specific. Using two electronic stethoscopes the examination takes place during opening and closing movements. That examination is safe for the patient and is easy even for inexperienced doctors. The measured signals from electronic stethoscopes are sent to the computer and the signals are analyzed [31].

3.2 Material and method

In our examination the patients with temporomandibular disorders were included based on our national version of The Research Diagnostic Criteria for Temporomandibular Disorders (RDC/TMD) as well as a group of patients without diagnoses but with symptoms and sounds from the joints region [32, 33]. After clinical examination, the auscultation procedure takes place. Patients with diagnoses based on RDC/TMD with sounds from temporomandibular joints and that those with joints sounds who did not receive the diagnoses were taken to the analyzes. All patients with other diagnoses without joints sounds were excluded from the study. After sound differentiation, the group suspected hypermobile joints were selected and an x-ray as confirmation was recommended.

3.2.1 Auscultation technic

Two electronic stethoscopes (Littmann Model 3200 Manufacturer 3 M Health Care, St. Paul, MN, USA) were used for the examination. Patients were asked to open and close the mouth 5 to 8 times. The auscultation of the temporomandibular joints region was carried out on both sides simultaneously. Electronic stethoscopes convert analogue signals to digital domains and make it possible to analyze about 15 s sounds. Stethoscopes provide a 4000 Hz sampling rate that ensures possibilities to reproduce sound components up to 2000 Hz. The measured sounds were sent to the computer to analyses the recorded signals. The representation of the signal in the frequency domain was computed with the use of the Numpy library and the fast

Fourier transform algorithm. In order to achieve local spectral representation, we split the signal into atomic sections with the Blackman window of 512 samples length and 256 samples overlapping. The frequencies below 80 Hz were removed from spectrograms to emphasize higher harmonics that were responsible for the effect of clicking [31]. Usage of two independent stethoscopes is beneficial in terms of capability of identification which joint generates sounds but on the other hand, makes difficulties in interpretation. Vibrations are conducted by bone and tissues therefore to differentiate where the origin of sound is located signals recorded by stethoscopes have to be synchronized. This feature is based on an external synchronization system. Small actuators placed on stethoscopes generate synchro beep sound and are triggered by physician during auscultation using a footswitch [34]. Promising results were achieved by signal analysis in time-frequency domain. This representation provides both information, when acoustic event occurred and which frequency components are present. Artificial intelligence-based approach seems to be the most appropriate in terms of mentioned signal analysis. Dedicated algorithms are still being developed. One of the main challenges is signal identification and segmentation [35]. Only when the auscultation signals will be split into parts corresponding to each jaw movement there will be possible to provide comprehensive automatic signals recognition algorithms.

3.3 Results

Totally 120 patients participated in the study. For sounds analyses were qualified 40 persons, in that group 32 were women. Hypermobile sounds were recognized in 4 patients (2 men and 2 women) based on lack of RDC/TMD diagnoses, sound analyses and x-ray confirmation.

From our research, we have very characteristic results for hypermobile joints in relation to the healthy one and with disk displacement with reduction, which is presented in **Figures 2–4**.

The sound record from a healthy temporomandibular joint presented in **Figure 2** concerns the time representation. The record representation is obtained from the serving program from electronic stethoscope Littmann 3200. It is worth mentioning that both joints do not present pathological sounds. Graphs represent a sound that indicates the correct movement of the structures of the temporomandibular joints during opening and closing.

In **Figure 3**, there is the signal representation from software Littmann 3200 from patient with disk displacement with reduction in both joints.

The signal time representation in **Figure 4** is characteristic for a person with subluxation in both joints.

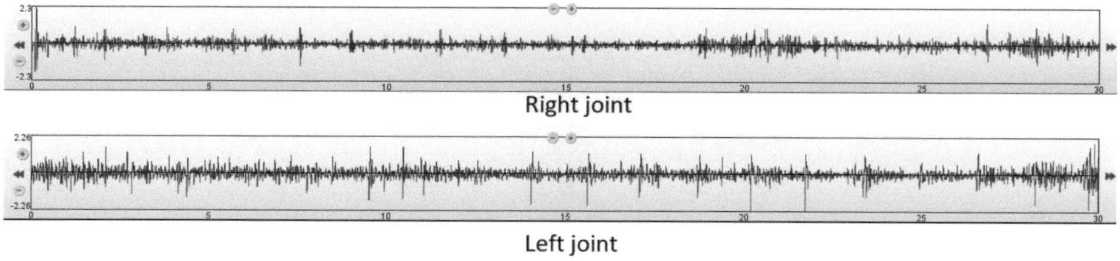

Figure 2.
The signal traces recorded on both sides in time domain in healthy joints.

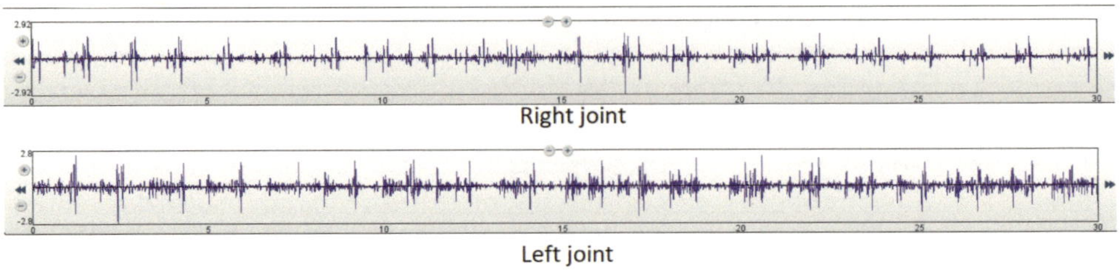

Figure 3.
The signal traces recorded on both sides in time domain from patients with disk displacement with reduction in both joints.

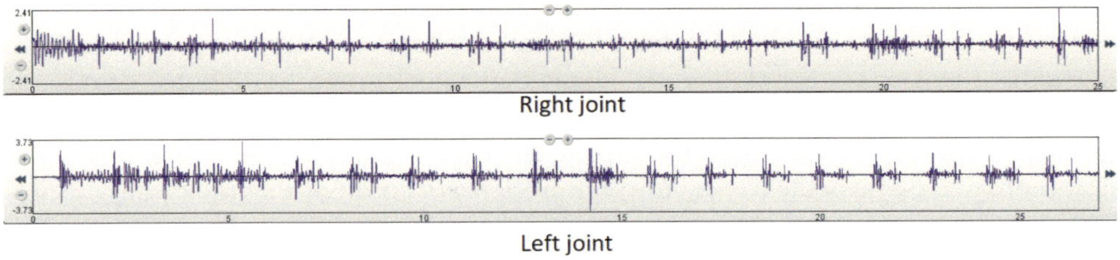

Figure 4.
The signal traces recorded on both sides in time domain from patients with hypermobile joints as subluxation.

Another helpful auscultation result is presented as time-frequency domain in the form of spectrograms (**Figures 5–7**).

As a complementary examination x-ray of the joints was required. The results are very characteristic in hypermobile jaw movements patients with a subluxation in one or both joints. For example, in **Figure 8** the position of the condyles in the front of the articular eminence was visible.

3.4 Discussion

The presented method of examination in the group of patients with temporomandibular joints region sounds is easy, inexpensive and gives possibility for future

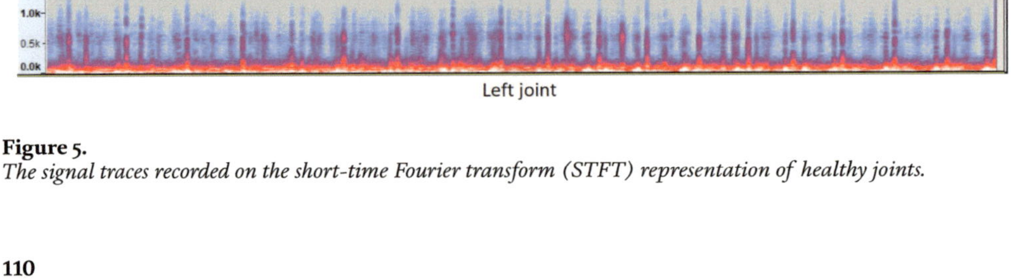

Figure 5.
The signal traces recorded on the short-time Fourier transform (STFT) representation of healthy joints.

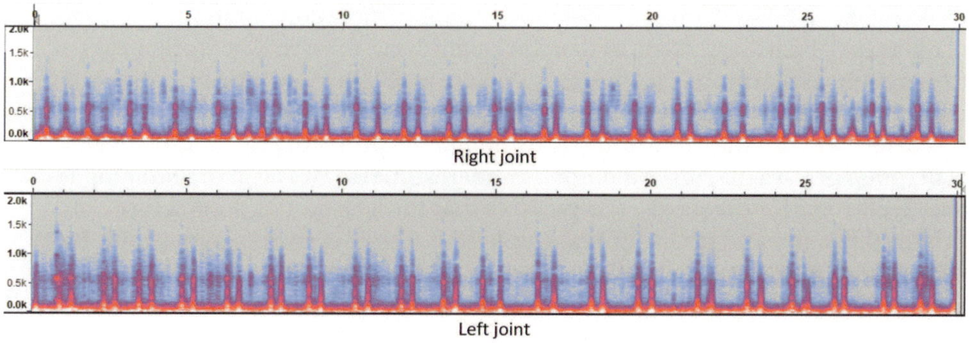

Figure 6.
The signal traces are recorded on the STFT representation of a disk displacement with reduction in both joints.

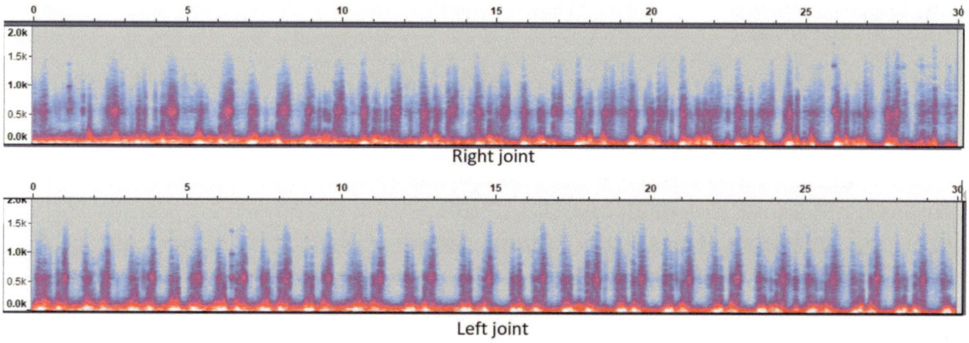

Figure 7.
Signal traces were recorded on the STFT representation of a hypermobile joints as subluxation.

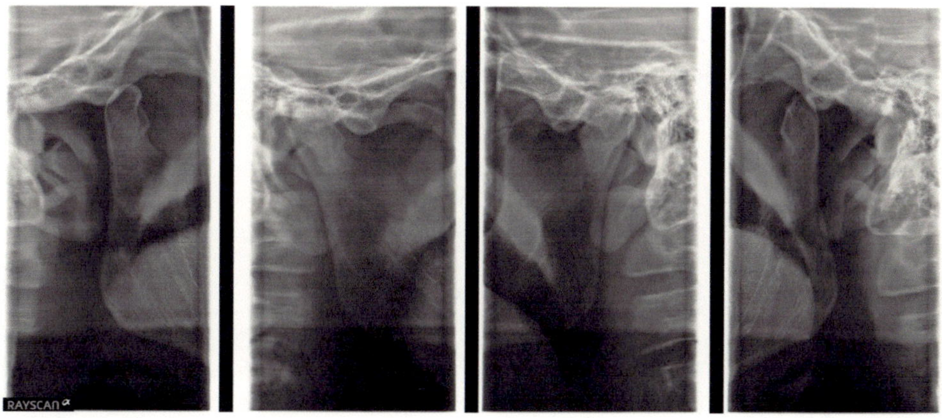

Figure 8.
An example of both sides subluxation x-ray. From left to right: Right side joint in wide jaw open position (the condyle head in the front of articular eminence), right side joint in maximal intercuspation position (the condyle head in glenoid fossa), left side joint in maximal intercuspation position (the condyle head in glenoid fossa) and left side joint in wide jaw open position (the condyle head in the front of articular eminence).

development. It takes the way for telemedicine as remote consultation. It allows enlargement of patients' medical data for monitoring present status and progress of treatment. Hypermobile jaw sounds are rare problem in a group of patients with temporomandibular disorders. In our group, it was 3.3% of examined patients which was correlated with the literature [2]. Although the problem affects a relatively small group of patients, it should not be underestimated. It is worth searching for simple solutions for diagnosis. It is possible that the lack of diagnosis is associated with the difficulty and no additional equipment. There is an alternative tool- BioJVA (BioResearch Associates, Inc. Milwaukee WI USA) that can be used to diagnose patients with temporomandibular disorders and for joints sounds analysis [36–38]. It is non-invasive diagnostic equipment, supplementing the basic clinical examination that can help to observe the present status and the effectiveness of the therapy. The use of this device is not common, it usually occurs in research medical centres due to very high prices and lack of knowledge of how to interpret diagnostic results. The use of a stethoscope could be a common examining method performed by every practising dentist.

4. Conclusion

As the summary about hypermobile temporomandibular jaw movements, it is important to know, that in all cases with subluxation the appearing sounds are frightening, and sometimes the doctors are more surprised than the accustomed patient. The associated unexpected jaw movements which are correlated with the thud sound in relation to inexperienced dentists would lead to a patient becoming sick. On the other hand, subluxation in some cases would lead to luxation and the patients may require surgery which is at risk of multiple complications. So the necessary recommendations for patients with hypermobile joints with the subluxation are to avoid wide mouth opening during yawning, eating or singing. The most difficult is to control jaw opening during yawning. Our recommendation is to bend your head to the chest and protect jaw opening by neck spine. Another possibility is to suction the tongue to the palate during yawning and protect wide opening by tongue frenulum. In addition, physiotherapeutic procedures are required, to strengthen the muscle for joints protection.

Author details

Jolanta E. Loster* and Justyna Grochala
Department of Prosthodontics and Orthodontics, Jagiellonian University in Kraków, Medical College, Dental Institute, Kraków, Poland

*Address all correspondence to: jolanta.loster@uj.edu.pl

References

[1] Prechel U, Ottl P, Ahlers OM, Neff A. The treatment of temporomandibular joint dislocation. Deutsches Arzteblatt International. 2018;**115**:59-64

[2] Marques-Mateo M, Puche-Torres M, Iglesias-Gimilio ME. Temporomandibular chronic dislocation: The long-standing condition. Medicina Oral, Patología Oral y Cirugía Bucal. 2016;**21**:e776-ee83

[3] Shorey CW, Campbell JH. Dislocation of the temporomandibular joint. Oral Surgery, Oral Medicine, Oral Pathology, Oral Radiology, and Endodontics. 2000;**89**:662-668

[4] Pogrel MA. Articular eminectomy for recurrent dislocation. The British Journal of Oral & Maxillofacial Surgery. 1987;**25**:237-243

[5] Akinbami BO. Evaluation of the mechanism and principles of management of temporomandibular joint dislocation. Systematic review of literature and a proposed new classification of temporomandibular joint dislocation. Head & Face Medicine. 2011;**7**:10

[6] The Glossary of Prosthodontic Terms Ninth Edition GPT-9. In: Ferro KJ, editor. The Journal of Prosthetic Dentistry. 2017;**117**:C1, e1-e105

[7] Beighton P, Horan F. Orthopaedic aspects of the Ehlers-Danlos syndrome. The Journal of Bone and Joint Surgery. British Volume. 1969;**51**:444-453

[8] Caminiti MF, Weinberg S. Chronic mandibular dislocation: The role of non-surgical and surgical treatment. Journal of the Canadian Dental Association. 1998;**64**:484-491

[9] Kai S, Kai H, Nakayama E, Tabata O, Tashiro H, Miyajima T, et al. Clinical symptoms of open lock position of the condyle. Relation to anterior dislocation of the temporomandibular joint. Oral Surgery, Oral Medicine, and Oral Pathology. 1992;**74**:143-148

[10] Merida-Velasco JR, Rodriguez JF, de la Cuadra C, Peces MD, Merida JA, Sanchez I. The posterior segment of the temporomandibular joint capsule and its anatomic relationship. Journal of Oral and Maxillofacial Surgery. 2007;**65**:30-33

[11] Slavicek R. *The Masticatory Organ*. Klosterneuburg: Gamma Medizinisch-wissenschaftliche Fortbildungs-GmbH; 2006

[12] Fernández Rubio EM, Radlanski RJ. Hypothesis for the lack of a muscular antagonist to the lateral pterygoid. Annals of Anatomy. Jan 2022;**239**:151841

[13] Schmolke C. The relationship between the temporomandibular joint capsule, articular disc and jaw muscles. Journal of Anatomy. 1994;**184**(Pt 2): 335-345

[14] Cheynet F, Guyot L, Richard O, Layoun W, Gola R. Discomallear and malleomandibular ligaments: Anatomical study and clinical applications. Surgical and Radiologic Anatomy: SRA. 2003;**25**:152-157

[15] Woodford SC, Robinson DL, Mehl A, Lee PVS, Ackland DC. Measurement of normal and pathological mandibular and temporomandibular joint kinematics: A systematic review. Journal of Biomechanics. 2020;**111**:109994

[16] Gross A, Bumann A, Hoffmeister B. Elastic fibers in the

human temporo-mandibular joint disc. International Journal of Oral and Maxillofacial Surgery. 1999;**28**:464-468

[17] Loster JE, Groch M, Wieczorek A, Muzalewska M, Skarka W. An evaluation of the relationship between the range of mandibular opening and the condyle positions in functional panoramic radiographs. Dental and Medical Problems. 2017;**54**:347-351

[18] Serrano-Hernanz G, Futarmal Kothari S, Castrillon E, Alvarez-Mendez AM, Ardizone-Garcia I, Svensson P. Importance of standardized palpationofthehumantemporomandibular joint. Journal of Oral & Facial Pain and Headache. 2019;**33**:220-226

[19] Schiffman E, Ohrbach R, Truelove E, Look J, Anderson G, Goulet JP, et al. Diagnosticcriteriafortemporomandibular disorders (DC/TMD) for clinical and research applications: Recommendations of the international RDC/TMD consortium network* and orofacial pain special interest Groupdagger. Journal of Oral & Facial Pain and Headache. 2014;**28**:6-27

[20] Mishutin EA, Geletin PN, Morozov VG. Audiodiagnostics in examination of patients with internal TMJ derangement. Stomatologiia. 2014;**93**:32-34

[21] Westling L, Helkimo E, Mattiasson A. Observer variation in functional examination of the temporomandibular joint. Journal of Craniomandibular Disorders: Facial & Oral Pain. 1992;**6**:202-207

[22] Dagar SR, Turakiya V, Pakhan AJ, Jaggi N, Kalra A, Vaidya V. Modified stethoscope for auscultation of temporomandibular joint sounds. Journal of International Oral Health: JIOH. 2014;**6**:40-44

[23] Widmalm SE, Williams WJ, Adams BS. The wave forms of temporomandibular joint sound clicking and crepitation. Journal of Oral Rehabilitation. 1996;**23**:44-49

[24] Emshoff R, Bertram S, Rudisch A, Gassner R. The diagnostic value of ultrasonography to determine the temporomandibular joint disk position. Oral Surgery, Oral Medicine, Oral Pathology, Oral Radiology, and Endodontics. 1997;**84**:688-696

[25] Limchaichana N, Nilsson H, Ekberg EC, Nilner M, Petersson A. Clinical diagnoses and MRI findings in patients with TMD pain. Journal of Oral Rehabilitation. 2007;**34**:237-245

[26] Westesson PL, Katzberg RW, Tallents RH, Sanchez-Woodworth RE, Svensson SA. CT and MR of the temporomandibular joint: Comparison with autopsy specimens. AJR. American Journal of Roentgenology. 1987;**148**:1165-1171

[27] Loster JE, Groch M, Ryniewicz WI, Osiewicz MA, Wieczorek A. Assessment of the range of mandibular movements as related to gender in polish young adult non-patients. Journal of Stomatology. 2016;**69**:146-152

[28] Bauss O, Sadat-Khonsari R, Fenske C, Engelke W, Schwestka-Polly R. Temporomandibular joint dysfunction in Marfan syndrome. Oral Surgery, Oral Medicine, Oral Pathology, Oral Radiology, and Endodontics. 2004;**97**:592-598

[29] Thexton A. A case of Ehlers-Danlos syndrome presenting with recurrent dislocation of the temporomandibular joint. The British Journal of Oral Surgery. 1965;**3**:190-193

[30] Osiewicz MA, Manfredini D, Loster BW, van Selms MKA, Lobbezoo F.

Comparison of the outcomes of dynamic/ static tests and palpation tests in TMD-pain patients. Journal of Oral Rehabilitation. 2018;**45**:185-190

[31] Grochala J, Grochala D, Kajor M, Iwaniec J, Loster JE, Iwaniec M. A novel method of temporomandibular joint hypermobility diagnosis based on signal analysis. Journal of Clinical Medicine. 2021;**10**

[32] Osiewicz MA, Lobbezoo F, Loster BW, Wilkosz M, Naeije M, Ohrbach R. Research diagnostic criteria for temporomandibular disorders (RDC/ TMD) - the polish version of a dual-axis system for the diagnosis of TMD. RDC/TMD form. Journal of Stomalogy. 2013;**66**:576-649

[33] Dworkin SF, LeResche L. Research diagnostic criteria for temporomandibular disorders: Review, criteria, examinations and specifications, critique. Journal of Craniomandibular Disorders: Facial & Oral Pain. 1992;**6**:301-355

[34] Lemejda J, Kajor M, Grochala D, Iwaniec M, Loster JE. Synchronous auscultation of temporomandibular joints using electronic stethoscopes. International Conference on Perspective Technologies and Methods in MEMS Design. 2020:146-149

[35] Djurdjanovic D, Widmalm SE, Williams WJ, Koh CK, Yang KP. Computerized classification of temporomandibular joint sounds. IEEE Transactions on Biomedical Engineering. 2000;**47**:977-984

[36] Radke J, Garcia R Jr, Ketcham R. Wavelet transforms of TM joint vibrations: A feature extraction tool for detecting reducing displaced disks. Cranio. 2001;**19**:84-90

[37] Kondrat W, Sierpińska T, Gołębiewska M. Vibration analysis of temporomandibular joints – BioJVA device description and its clinical application in dental diagnostics – Review of literature. Journal of Stomatology. 2012;**65**:207-215

[38] Kondrat W, Sierpinska T, Radke J. Assessment of the temporomandibular joint function in young adults without complaints from the masticatory system. International Journal of Medical Sciences. 2018;**15**:161-169

Chapter 9

Temporomandibular Joint Pain

Kadarkarai Kirupa, R. Rajashri, Kamali Raman, Aishwarya Balaji, Pavithra Elango, Swetha Karupaiah and Leelavathy Gopalakrishnan

Abstract

Temporomandibular joint (TMJ) is a synovial articulation between mandibular condyle and glenoid fossa in the temporal bone. Any structural and/or functional changes can affect the TMJ and related structures. Temporomandibular disorder (TMD) is a heterogeneous group of musculoskeletal disorders mainly characterised by regional pain in the facial and preauricular area and/or limitations/interference of jaw movement. TMD has multifactorial aetiology, which includes biology, and environmental social, emotional, and cognitive factors. TMD is more common orofacial pain condition and nondental origin. Factors associated with TMD include other pain condition, auto-immune disorder and psychiatric illness. The clinical conditions may present with limitation in opening and closing mouth, pain and articular noise. So this chapter mainly deals with the classification of TMJ disorder, diagnosis and management particularly TENS and ultrasound therapy for TMJ disorder.

Keywords: temporomandibular joint, TMJ disorders, TENS, pain, ultrasound therapy

1. Introduction

The temporomandibular joint (TMJ) is a synovial joint. The joint is the articulation between the mandibular condyle and the glenoid fossa in the temporal bone. Temporomandibular joint disorders produce structural and functional changes of the joint. Temporalis, medial & lateral pterygoid, Masseter Maxilla/upper jaw Mandible/lower jaw and the temporal. These disorders may present with specific clinical features such as pain, muscle tightness, limitation in opening and closing the mouth [1].

TMJ is the most complex joint. TMJ disorders occur when the muscles, ligament, joint capsule or any other structure surrounding the TMJ joint are affected. This consists of joint cavity, mandibular condyle, articular disc, muscle and nerve, which interacts with various structures such as cervical spine and orofacial region. When the physiological functions of some of these components are altered, functional and structural disorders result in clinical impact [2]. The unique feature of TMJ is that it acts as a fulcrum in which the movement is controlled by both morphology of joints and the dentition at the other end.

During life, the components of the joints including temporal, condylar and disc articular surfaces undergo continuous remodelling. The synovial fluid is responsible for nourishment and lubrication. The lateral pterygoid muscle is attached to the joint capsule. The function of the articular disc is to produce friction, stabilisation and viscoelastic properties. Mastication and speech are the main action of TMJ joint [3].

During mastication process, this joint supports a large number of forces. Excessive force on the joint can cause damage in its structure or alter normal function contact of condyles, discs and eminence. This damage and alteration can result in pain, dysfunction or both [3].

Temporomandibular disorders (TMDs) are group of heterogeneous musculoskeletal disorders mainly responsible for regional pain in the facial and preauricular, limitation and interference of the jaw movements. TMD has many causes, which includes biologic, environmental, social, emotional and cognitive factors. Factors associated with TMD include other pain condition (e.g. chronic headaches, fibromyalgia), autoimmune disorders, sleep apnoea and psychiatric illness. TMDs are the most common orofacial pain conditions other than dental origin [4].

Numerous risk factors have been implicated including joint and muscle trauma, anatomical factors (e.g. skeletal and occlusal relationship), pathophysiological factors (e.g. bone and connective tissue disorders, sensitization of peripheral and CNS pain processing pathways) and psychosocial factors (e.g. depression and anxiety, emotional and perceptual responses to psychological stressors).

2. Prevalences

The prevalence of TMDs is around 12% of world population and 35 million people in US. TMDs affect both men and women but majority seeking care are women of age group 19–49 years. TMD is diagnosed in women 2–5 times more frequently than men. Studies suggest that women tend to have more severe symptoms and are nine times as likely to be diagnosed with majority limitations in jaw movements and unremitting pain.

There are various hypothesis put forward by several researchers to demonstrate the higher prevalence rate in women. Anatomical, hormonal, behavioural and genetic differences contribute to the disproportional ratio of women to men diagnosed [4].

Anatomical differences between males and females in jaw and skull affect the forces on TMJ. Maxillary bone is longer, wider and thicker in males than in females. The angle created by mandible is less obtuse in male than in female. Mandibular condyle is larger and temporal socket is deeper in males. All these anatomical factors create more stable environment for TMJ translation in males than in females.

Hormonal differences between men and women contribute to TMDs. Oestrogen and progesterone levels are higher in women during childbearing years. There is increased ligament laxity during preovulatory phase (oestrogen dominates). During follicular phase (days 1–9), relaxin hormone is secreted and it peaks during the luteal phase (days 15–28). These differences in the level of hormones released may contribute to greater laxity in some women. Increased ligament laxity increases joint play and it irritates the joints.

Behavioural differences—Men and women manage stress differently. Clenching, grinding and poor breathing habits can increase internalisation of stress and it may irritate TMJ [5].

Various studies revealed that at least one sign of articular dysfunction is seen in about 40–75% of cases in general adult population, and in 33% of cases, there is at least one symptom of dysfunction. Signs such as noise and asymmetric mouth opening are prevalent in about 50% of the individuals and other symptoms such as difficulty in mouth opening are present in about 5% of cases [6]. Articular disorders are present in 19%, muscular forms of disorders in 23% and both in 27% of individuals in general population. In patients, these symptoms are more pronounced in 20–40 age group, and in general population, these symptoms are most commonly seen in 17–30 age groups.

Prevalence of moderate or severe TMDs was found to be 37.4% in children and adolescents between 6 and 14 years of age in Brazilian study.

Epidemiological surveys reported that 50–70% of population have signs of a disorder at some stage during their life, whereas an estimated 20–25% of the population have symptoms of TMD. The highest prevalence of TMD in relation to age has been estimated between the age of 20 and 40s. Among the post-menopausal women, those receiving hormone replacement therapy (HRT) were found to be at higher risk for TMD than those not receiving HRT. TMD is most prevalent in adolescents and women during the reproductive years and falls off sharply with advancing middle age [7].

3. Classification of TMJ disorders

The temporomandibular joint is mainly classified into three main groups:

GROUP I—MUSCLE DISORDERS.

GROUP II—ARTHRALGIA, ARTHRITIS & ARTHROSIS.

GROUP III—DISC DISPLACEMENT.

Group I consist of myofascial pain and myofascial pain with limitation in aperture.

Group II consists of arthralgia (joint pain), osteoarthritis and osteoarthrosis.

Group III consists of disc displacement with reduction, disc limitation without reduction, and disc displacement without reduction and with limitation of aperture.

TMD can be further subdivided into pain-related disorders such as myofascial pain and arthralgia and typically non-painful disorders.

TMDs are characterised by pain in the preauricular area, TMJ/muscles of mastication, limitation/deviation in the mandibular ROM and TMJ sounds (clicking, popping and crepitus) during mandibular function, headaches and jaw tenderness on function. Clicking is the most common symptom of TMJ dysfunction.

A number of studies have examined physical therapy for TMJ dysfunction and pain, including massage, electrotherapy, active exercise and manipulation therapy. Ultrasound therapy reduces pain and inflammation and improves mouth function [8].

3.1 Causes

The main causes Of TMJ disorder are unclear, but it is multifactorial.

Capsule inflammation and muscle pain are caused by occlusion, stress, anxiety or abnormalities of intra-articular disk. Parafunctional habits may cause TMJ micro-trauma or masticatory muscle hyperactivity [9].

TMJ disorders may also arise after macro-trauma or facial trauma also due to malposition of TMJ disc termed 'internal derangement' and osteoarthritic changes.

Severely injured in the TMJ leads to disordered; for example, it can result in a severe blow on the jaw to break bones or damaged disk, which could destroy the smooth movement of the joint, causing pain or bad occlusion [10].

Some behavioural factors like continuous chewing gum may also lead to unrest in the TMJ joint.

3.2 Clinical features

Joint erosion, osteophyte formation, hypoplasia, subchondral cyst, flattening of articular eminence and reduced jaw movements were seen.

Worsened mastication was common findings in temporomandibular joint Osteoarthritis (TMJ-OA).

General pain was correlated with condylar flattening.

Masticatory efficiency correlates with condylar flattening and sclerosis.

Psychological features like Bruxism, sleep disturbances, anxiety and depression will be seen [11].

Jaws are used to lock while opening or closing the mouth.

Head ache.

Tooth pain.

Lack of facial expression mainly over the lower face.

Pain in the neck and shoulders.

Difficulty in chewing [12].

3.3 Diagnosis

Along with proper clinical examination, imaging of TMJ joint is also necessary. The most common methods are computed tomography (CT) and magnetic resonance imaging (MRI). Even though it has many advantages, it suffers certain drawbacks, being expensive, having necessity of advanced equipment, longer time needed to use it for TMJ images, its restricted use in patients with claustrophobia, pacemakers and metallic prosthesis.

Ultrasonography has been suggested as an alternative diagnostic method in the imaging of TMJ disorders, because it is less expensive.

High-resolution ultrasonography (HR-US) is the best way to investigate the TMJ conditions. The articular disk can be clearly seen during the mouth opening movement [13].

3.3.1 Differential diagnosis

- Dental pain
- Referred pain—sinuses, ear, nose, cervical disease, systemic
- Neuralgias, neurologic pain disorders
- Central lesions
- Somatoform disorders
- Disorders of the temporomandibular
- Eagle's syndrome
- Maxillary sinusitis
- Management for temperomandibular joint disorders.

3.4 Ultrasound

TMD is one of the most common causes of pain in the mouth and face, affecting millions of people. It often leads to chronic pain that lasts for years. The physiotherapy management of TMJ joints includes massage, exercise and modalities. Modalities mainly the TENS and ULTRASOUND have proven to reduce pain and other symptoms of the TMJ joint disorders [14].

However, the prognosis of the treatment is relatively slow in relieving pain for patients. Ultrasound (US) has been used for treating temporomandibular joint Osteoarthritis (TMJ-OA) and hypoxia-induced chondrocytes damage in TMDs.

The ultrasound mechanical vibration is transmitted into the body as high-frequency acoustic pressure waves. These waves will mechanically stimulate living tissues, resulting in tissue healing. The ultrasound will promote cell proliferation and the synthesis of extracellular matrix in fibroblasts and myoblasts, which eventually reduces inflammation and promotes regeneration in various injured soft tissues [15].

4. Technique

Direct bath method

The treatment area should be clear and flat. Then, the coupling medium like aquasonic gel should be applied to prevent excess air between the skin and treatment head and to allow the ultrasonic beam to pass through the body tissues. The treatment head is moved in rhythmic direction in order to avoid concentration at one point.

Parameters

- FREQUENCY-3MHZ (superficial) or 1MHZ (deeper)
- INTENSITY-0.8–1 W/cm^2
- MODE-Continuous mode
- DURATION-3 minutes

Thermal effects

- Absorption of tissues
- The efficiency of circulation through the insonated tissues
- When using continuous ultrasound, the amount of heat developed is directly proportional to the intensity and duration of insonation.

Nonthermal effects

- **Cavitation** is the oscillatory activity of highly compressible bodies within the tissues such as gas- or vapour-filled voids.

It may be **stable** or **unstable** cavitation.

- **Stable cavitation** occurs when bubbles oscillate to and fro within the ultrasonic pressure waves but remains intact. And it modifies the ultrasonic beam in such a way so as to cause micro-streaming.

- **Unstable cavitation** occurs when the volume of the bubbles rapidly then collapses. It is potentially dangerous to the tissues as the collapse of the bubbles causes a great local rise in temperature. It is avoided by moving the treatment head using a low intensity.

- **Micro-massage** occurs where the longitudinal compression waves of the ultrasound beam produce compression and rarefaction of the cells and affect the movement of tissue fluid in interstitial spaces. This can help in reducing oedema

- **Biological effect** helps to clear the area of debris and to increase the tensile strength of the scar by affecting the direction, strength and elasticity of fibres [16].

5. Discussion

Ultrasound is defined as sound frequency 20,000 cycles per second. Ultrasound travels through materials. It is the modality that is used for a number of purposes including diagnosis destruction of tissue and therapy. Ultrasonic energy generated at 1MHZ is transmitted through the more superficial tissues and absorbed primarily in the deeper tissue at depths of 3-5 cm. Patient should be in lying position with head support with pillow in continuous mode with duration of 5 to 8 min. The treatment head is moved continuously over the surface, while even pressure is maintained in order to iron out irregularities in sonic field. The pattern of movement can be series of overlapping parallel strokes, circles or figure of eight. The effect of ultrasound increases intracellular ca, increases skin and membrane permeability, increases macrophage response, promotes healing, reduces swelling, and increases blood flow.

Many studies recommend ultrasound is effective for TMD treatment. The beneficial effect of Ultrasound may be associated with the effect of micro-destruction. In addition to reduction of pain in TMJ treatment, ultrasound treatment shows improvement in jaw functions.

The therapeutic effect is persistent in follow-up period of 6 months with less than 3% recurrence rate after ultrasound treatment; therefore, ultrasound may be recommended for TMD treatment [17].

Shuang Ba et al. concluded that US has been shown to be able to reduce excessive cytokine content in the articular fluid and the apoptosis of chondrocytes. It promotes the proliferation of articular cartilage to repair cartilage defects and inhibits the secretion of inflammatory cytokines. Hence, treating by ultrasound reduces pain effectively [18].

Sanyuktha et al. state that the generated heat presumed to increase tissue cell metabolism, which in turn helps to promote soft tissue healing. The sound wave causes tissue vibration creating heat in the treatment field and thus increases the blood flow. The pain reduces with the resolution of information.

Zhou et al. explored the efficacy of US in terms of mandibular condylar cartilage repair *via* autophagy regulation. And it reduced the injury severity and upregulated the autophagy biomarkers [19].

Liang et al. stated that US has decreased the proliferation of chondrocytes and increased the osteoclast activity in the calcified cartilage layer [20].

6. TMJ management (TENS)

Only 5–10% of patients require treatment for TMD, and 40% of patients have spontaneous resolutions of symptoms. In a long-term follow-up study, 50–90% of patients had pain relief after conservative therapy. There is evidence that supports the use of physical therapy for improving symptoms associated with TMD. TENS is one of such treatment modalities that merit unique consideration and it is one of the safest and most inexpensive modalities that are used to control both chronic and acute pains.

TENS FOR TMJ

TENS is a well-known physical therapy, which is useful for the relief of pain. Transcutaneous electrical nerve stimulation (TENS) is one of the most effective physical therapy techniques. TENS is the application of low-frequency current in form of pulsed rectangular currents through surface electrodes on the patient's skin to reduce pain.

Principles

TENS works on the principle that electrical stimulation is directed to pain areas *via* surface electrodes, and current passes through these areas, which reduces or eliminates pain. It is safe and non-invasive and effective method. Electrodes made of silicon are used for TENS. They are placed at the area with the highest pain, in the same dermatome, myotomes and/or myofascial trigger points. They can also be placed on the course or on the supplied muscles of the corresponding peripheral nerve.

Patient's position: sitting.
Therapist position: standing behind the patient.
Method: direct method.
Electrode placement: TM joint and nape of neck.
Pulse duration: 50–200 μs.
Frequency: 50 mA–100 mA.
Duration: 15 min.

7. Effects and uses

Effect of TENS is based on gate control theory and pain modulation.

TENS stimulates thick, myelinated, sensory fibres (A-fibres), which in turn blocks the impulses of pain-modulating fibres (C-fibres) and closes the gate to pain signals at the level of their entry into the spinal cord. In TENS, low-frequency and high-intensity or high-frequency and low-intensity electrical stimulation is applied, it gives sharp stimulus carried towards cerebellum, and its passage through the midbrain will cause the periaqueductal area of grey matter and raphe nuclei to interact to release opiate-like substance at cord level. The enkephalins and endorphins released have the effect of blocking forward transmission in the pain circuit. TENS treatment also relaxes the jaw muscles, lesser the degree of stress, and reduces the pain [21].

According to the gate control theory, when the large diameter, low-threshold mechanoreceptors are stimulated by simple mechanical stimulation of the receptors in the skin, muscle or joints or by electrical stimulation, the SG cells are stimulated through an excitatory synapse. The SG cells, receiving inputs from nociceptors and mechanoreceptors, integrates and modulates the pain fiber activity and prevents transmission of nociceptive information to higher centers.

8. Discussion

Rathi Rela et al. also concluded that TENS therapy showed favourable results in pain management in TMD patient [22].

Y. Zhang et al. state that TENS could attenuate movement-evoked pain and improve jaw motor function during repeated jaw movements. This study indicated that movement-evoked pain was reduced either spontaneously or by TENS in TMJ pain patients [23].

G.moger et al. concluded that TENS shows good results in relieving muscular pain and chronic pain [24].

The useful effects of the TENS are explained by different theories. One theory is that TENS directly stimulate the motor nerves resulting in rhythmic contraction of the masticator muscles. These changes lead to increased blood flow and oxygen to the muscles, and reduce interstitial oedema and build-up of harmful toxins. Thus, overall result is reduction of pain and improved mobility of TMJ.

Instead of pain, your brain feels the pleasant tingling, massage-like sensation of the TENS, and the TENS current also stimulates your body to produce endorphin, which creates dull pain and sense of well-being.

TENS treatment also relaxes the jaw muscles, lesser the degree of stress, and reduces the pain.

Acknowledgements

I would like to thank the FOUNDER CHANCELLOR THIRU Dr. A.C. SHANMUGAM, B.A., B.L., PRESIDENT Er. A.C.A. ARUN KUMAR B. Tech, MBA., SECRETARY THIRU A. RAVI KUMAR MBA., and VICE CHANCELLOR Prof. Dr. S. GEETHA LAKSHMI MBBS., MD., PhD.

I would like to express my sincere gratitude to my PRINCIPAL Prof. Dr. C.V. SENTHIL NATHAN, MPT (geriatrics), PGDDR, M.I.A.P., MHPC, MISCP, VICE PRINICIPAL Dr. V. RAJALAKSHMI, MPT (Neuro), PhD and Dr. S. VEENA @ KRITHIKA, MPT (Neuro), PhD.

Author details

Kadarkarai Kirupa*, R. Rajashri, Kamali Raman, Aishwarya Balaji, Pavithra Elango, Swetha Karupaiah and Leelavathy Gopalakrishnan
DR. M.G.R. Education and Research Institute, India

*Address all correspondence to: kirupa.physio@drmgrdu.ac.in

References

[1] Solak Ö, Turhan-Haktanır N, Köken G, et al. Prevalence of temporomandibular disorders in pregnancy. European Journal of General Medicine. 2009;**6**(4):223-228

[2] AlShaban KK, Gul Abdul Waheed Z. Prevalence of TMJ disorders among the patients attending the Dental Clinic of Ajman University of Science and Technology-Fujairah Campus, UAE. International Journal of Dentistry. 2018;**2018**:9861623. DOI: 10.1155\2018\98616232. PMID: 29861731. PMCID: PMC5971318

[3] Gopal SK, Shankar SR, Vardhan BGH. Prevalence of temporo-mandibular joint disorders in symptomatic and asymptomatic patients: A cross-sectional study. International Journal of Advanced Science. 2014;**1**:14-20

[4] Poveda-Roda R, Bagan JV, Diaz-Fernandez JM, Hernandez-Bazan S, Jimenez-Soriano Y. Review of temporomandibular joint pathology. Part of temporomandibular joint pathology. Part I: Classification, epidemiology and risk factors. Medicina Oral, Patologia Oral Y Cirugia Bucal. 2007;**12**:E292-E298

[5] American Academy of Pediatric Dentistry. Acquired Temporomandibular Disorders in Infants, Children, and Adolescents. The Reference Manual of Pediatric Dentistry. Chicago, Ill: American Academy of Pediatric Dentistry; 2021

[6] Shet RG, Rao S, Patel R, Suvvati P, Sadar LR, Yadav RD. Prevalence of temporomandibular joint dysfunction and its signs among the partially edentulous patients in a village of North Gujarat. The Journal of Contemporary Dental Practice. 2013;14(6):1151

[7] Herb K, Cho S, Stiles MA. Temporomandibular joint pain and dysfunction. Current Pain and Headache Reports. 2006;**10**(6):408-414

[8] Durham J, Newton-John TR, Zakrzewska JM. Temporomandibular disorders. BMJ. 2015;**350**:h1154

[9] Zakrzewska JM. Temporomandibular disorders, headaches and chronic pain. Journal of Pain & Palliative Care Pharmacotherapy. 2015;**29**(1):61-63

[10] Schiffman E, Ohrbach R, Truelove E, et al. Diagnostic criteria for temporomandibular disorders (DC/TMD) for clinical and research applications: Recommendations of the international RDC/TMD consortium network and orofacial pain special interest groupdagger. Journal of Oral & Facial Pain and Headache. 2014;**28**(1):6

[11] Miernik M, Wieckiewicz M, Paradowska A, Wieckiewicz W. Massage therapy in myofascial TMD pain management. Advances in Clinical and Experimental Medicine. 2012;**21**(5):681-685

[12] Morell GC. Manual therapy improved signs and symptoms of temporomandibular disorders. Evidence-Based Dentistry. 2016;**17**(1):25-26

[13] Bevilaqua-Grosso D, Monteiro-Pedro V, Guirro RR, Berzin F. A physiotherapeutic approach to craniomandibular disorders: A case report. Journal of Oral Rehabilitation. 2002;**29**(3):268-273

[14] Sanders C, Liegey-Dougall A, Haggard R, et al. Temporomandibular disorder diagnostic groups affect outcomes independently of treatment in

patients at risk for developing chronicity: A 2-year follow-up study. Journal of Oral & Facial Pain and Headache. 2016;**30**(3): 187-202

[15] Zhou FH, Zhao HY. Acupuncture and ultrasound therapy for temporomandibular disorders. Di Yi Jun Yi Da XueXueBao. 2004;**24**(6):720-721

[16] Kraus M, Reinhart E, Krause H, Reuther J. Low energy extracorporeal shockwave therapy (ESWT) for treatment of myogelosis of the masseter muscle. Mund-, Kiefer- und Gesichtschirurgie. 1999;**3**(1):20-23

[17] Rodrigues D, Oliveira AS, Bérzin F. Effect of conventional TENS on pain and electromyographic activity of masticatory muscles in TMD patients. Brazilian Oral Research. 2004;**18**(4):290-295

[18] Tanaka E, Liu Y, Xia L, et al. Effectiveness of low-intensity pulsed ultrasound on osteoarthritis of the temporomandibular joint: A review. Annals of Biomedical Engineering. 2020;**48**(8):2158-2170

[19] Garefis P, Grigoriadou E, Zarifi A, et al. Effectiveness of conservative treatment for craniomandibular disorders: A 2-year longitudinal study. Journal of Orofacial Pain. 1994;**8**(3):309-314

[20] Indresano A, Alpha C. Nonsurgical management of temporomandibular joint disorders. In: Fonseca RJ, Marciani RD, Turvey TA, editors. Oral and Maxillofacial Surgery. 2nd ed. St. Louis, Mo: Saunders/Elsevier; 2009. pp. 881-897

[21] Esposito CJ, Shay JS, Morgan B. Electronic dental anesthesia: A pilot study. Quintessence International. 1993;**24**(3):167-170

[22] Walsh DM, Howe TE, Johnson MI, et al. Transcutaneous electrical nerve stimulation for acute pain. Cochrane Database of Systematic Reviews. 2009;**2**(Art. N):CD006142

[23] Cooper BC. The role of bioelectronic instruments in the management of TMD. The New York State Dental Journal. 1995;**61**(9):48-53

[24] Gomez CE, Christensen LV. Stimulus-response latencies of two instruments delivering transcutaneous electrical neuromuscular stimulation (TENS). Journal of Oral Rehabilitation. 1991;**18**(1):87-94